Games for Health 2014

Ben Schouten · Stephen Fedtke ·
Marlies Schijven · Mirjam Vosmeer ·
Alex Gekker
Editors

Games for Health 2014

Proceedings of the 4th conference on
gaming and playful interaction in
healthcare

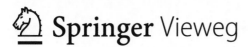 Springer Vieweg

Editors

Ben Schouten
Department of Industrial Design
Eindhoven University of Technology
Eindhoven, Netherlands

Stephen Fedtke
Zug, Switzerland

Marlies Schijven
Department of Surgery
Academic Medical Center Amsterdam
Amsterdam, Netherlands

Mirjam Vosmeer
Amsterdam University of Applied Sciences
Amsterdam, Netherlands

Alex Gekker
Utrecht University
Utrecht, Netherlands

ISBN 978-3-658-07140-0   ISBN 978-3-658-07141-7 (eBook)
DOI 10.1007/978-3-658-07141-7

Library of Congress Control Number: 2014951225

Springer Vieweg

Printed on acid-free paper

Springer Vieweg is a brand of Springer DE. Springer DE is part of Springer Science+Business Media.
www.springer-vieweg.de

Preface

The Fourth European Games for Health Conference 2014 (GFHEU 2014) brings together researchers, medical professionals and game developers to share information about the impact of games, playful interaction and game technologies on health, health care and health policy. Over two days, more than 500 attendees will participate, in over 13 sessions provided by an international array of more than 50 speakers, cutting across a wide range of activities in health and well-being. Conference topics include exergaming, physical therapy, disease management, health behaviour change, biofeedback, scientific validation, rehab, epidemiology, training, cognitive health, nutrition and education.

As we are aiming for innovation and further integration of research and game development in health care, this year we continued to add an extra academic track to the conference. These proceedings are the outcome of that integration and contain 20 full papers presented at the conference in the form of oral presentations or posters. In this volume we have opted for not breaking down the papers into separate chapters. Our previous experience has taught us that such divisions are always a bit artificial, and so much more when dealing with health games. The academic track is interwoven into the conference's broader structure to further promote dialogue between academics and practitioners working within the fields of Game & Play Studies, Design Research, Game Development and the Medical Community, exploring and innovating within the greater area of health. This track is labelled 'Share your Research' in your conference program.

Yet, looking over the works submitted to this volume, few interesting trends are discerned.

Social relatedness and empowerment of the (end) user
Not always following the predominately-paternalistic approach, health games aim to facilitate self-efficacy and allow people to take charge of their own health and wellbeing. Designers and doctors join together to empower the patients like never before. Games are not only regarded as products (applications) but also as services for a longstanding relationship between patients, doctors, relatives and care providers or between medical doctors and students, to learn the practice of medicine. Several papers in these proceedings address motivational issues and meaningful (adaptive) feedback to facilitate these longstanding relationships. Moreover it becomes practice to integrate the game, app or applied toy in already existing forms of therapy, educational practices or other application domains. Using the gaming's affinity with social play and the rising spreadability of media over social networking sites, the focus shifts from top-down to bottom-up and more participatory healthcare.

Theory and educational practice.
The theory of games for health in health care settings is also gaining traction, such as modelling patients behaviour in clinical immersive environments targeting at medical education or the theoretical underpinning of exergames. Perhaps even more

important is to study the public acceptance of these applications, allowing the game designer to anticipate in the design of even better appreciated games and play experiences. A clear trend, happily supported by the Games4Health conference, is the increase of number of games used in professional education of medical doctors.

Game mechanics, architecture and data.

Digital games allow players to use advanced computational power, (haptic) devices, consoles, wearable's, visualization, persuasive technology and create immersive environments. Using the Oculus Rift in games for pain management is a good example, but also adaptive games that take into account the abilities of the individual players. As health games become further embedded in the toolsets of caretakers and patients alike, a call for standardization and new architectures arises. Whether in the form of building rigid data structures to share between platforms, or more particular recommendations for world-builders, the call for agreed frameworks is out there.

Validation.

As always, validation is a hot topic, but perhaps an interesting trend is emerging in coupling validation with design theory. No longer based on traditional validation techniques originating purely in the medical domain, validation through design is the next thing. Which means that a therapy, cure or rehabilitation can be validated on its effect but also can be used to evaluate and deepen the design (theory of) the game mechanics.

In view of this all, the GFHEU 2014 proceedings can be considered as a timely document that provides many new results and insights in the new field of Games for Health. We would like to thank all members of the Program Committee for their most valuable and highly appreciated contribution to the conference by reading submissions, writing reviews, and participating in the discussion phase. We hope to provide you with many pleasant and fruitful reading hours.

August 2014   Ben Schouten
Amsterdam   Chair Program Committee

Organization

Organizing Committee

Conference Chair:
> Jurriaan van Rijswijk (Games for Health Europe)

Program Chair
> Ben Schouten (Eindhoven University of Technology)

Organizers
> Hannieta Beuving (Games for Health Europe)
> Alex Gekker (University of Utrecht)
> Sandra van Rijswijk (Games for Health Europe)

Reviewers

Albert Salah	Bogazici University, Istanbul, Turkey
Alex Gekker	University of Utrecht & Games for Health Europe, Netherlands
Bart Brandenburg	Medicinfo, Netherlands
Ben Schouten	Eindhoven University of Technology & Amsterdam University of Applied Sciences, Netherlands
Berry Eggen	Eindhoven University of Technology, Netherlands
David Nieborg	University of Amsterdam, Netherlands.
Ellis Bartholomeus	Ellisinwonderland, Netherlands
Erik Van Der Spek	Eindhoven University of Technology, Netherlands
Erinc Salor	University of Amsterdam, Netherlands.
Joris Dormans	Amsterdam University of Applied Sciences, Netherlands.
Marcelo Vasconcellos	Oswaldo Cruz Foundation – Fiocruz, Brazil
Marlies Schijven	Academic Medical Center Amsterdam, Netherlands.
Matthias Rauterberg	Eindhoven University of Technology, Netherlands
Mirjam Vosmeer	Amsterdam University of Applied Sciences, Netherlands.
Rafael Bidarra	Delft University of Technology, Netherlands.
Simon McCallum	Gjøvik University College, Norway
Stephanie Klein Nagelvoort-Schuit	Erasmus University, Rotterdam, Netherlands
Vero Vanden Abeele	eMedia Lab, Group T – Leuven Engineering School, CUO Catholic University Leuven, Belgium.

Table of Contents

Table of Contents

"On call: antibiotics"- development and evaluation of a serious antimicrobial prescribing game for hospital care

Enrique Castro-Sánchez[1], Esmita Charani[1], Luke SP Moore[1], Myriam Gharbi[1],
and Alison H Holmes[1]

[1]National Institute for Health Research Health Protection Research Unit (NIHR HPRU)
in Healthcare Associated Infection and Antimicrobial Resistance at Imperial College London,
London, United Kingdom
{e.castro-sanchez, e.charani, l.moore, m.gharbi,
alison.holmes}@imperial.ac.uk

Abstract: Improved antimicrobial prescribing is a key effort to reduce the impact of increasing antimicrobial resistance. Quality improvement programmes in antimicrobial prescribing have to ensure the continued engagement of prescribers with optimal prescribing behaviours. Serious games have been proposed to improve clinical practice and may serve to resolve some of the behavioural and social barriers influencing prescribing. We describe here the ongoing development and future evaluation of a mobile device-based serious antimicrobial prescribing game for hospital clinicians.

Keywords: antimicrobial prescribing, antimicrobial stewardship, serious game, gamification

1   Introduction

Increasing antimicrobial resistance has been identified as a global threat to health [1]. Antimicrobial stewardship, or the prudent use of antimicrobials, has been advocated to arrest the advance of resistance [2]. A variety of antimicrobial stewardship measures have been implemented with varying success rates to improve the quality of antimicrobial prescribing. Whilst prescriber knowledge and skills are important, attention to behavioural and social aspects in prescribing appear equally essential to sustain improvement initiatives [3]. Serious games have been used to provide effective interactive learning and practice in surgery [4], as well as for undergraduate medical education [5]. The use of psychological techniques used in games ('gamification') has also been successfully introduced in other clinical settings to maintain clinicians' commitment to desired behaviours [6], prolonging the sustainability of quality improvement programmes and resolving some of the issues related to engagement affecting traditional intervention. The National Centre for Infection Prevention and Management (CIPM) at Imperial College London had previously developed successful smartphone apps focused on local antibiotic prescribing policies, highlighting the potential for electronic and mobile technologies to fill the gap between information provision and behaviour change [7].

1

2   Objectives

We proposed the development of a serious prescribing game for computers and portable devices to support and encourage the prudent use of antimicrobials in hospitals prescribers. The development and evaluation of the serious prescribing game was our primary objective. Additionally, exploring the uptake, acceptability, and utility of the game as a tool to modify the behaviour of prescribing clinicians were some of the secondary objectives.

3   Materials and methods

The game is powered by a Unity game engine (Unity Technologies, USA), allowing for portability and multiplatform compatibility. Thus, the current game build can be installed and played in PC and Mac computers, as well as Android and iOS smartphone and tablet devices. We endeavoured to develop a product with light system requirements, in view of the potential for deployment and use in low- and middle-income countries.

3.1   Clinical elements

A series of virtual patients (Figure 1) were prepared in collaboration with commercial game developers, designers and clinicians (including doctors, pharmacists and nurses). These cases allowed clinicians to practice prescribing behaviours in a simulated environment, understanding the steps involved in the prescribing process and gaining a comprehensive overview of their professional role and the impact of antimicrobial prescribing decisions in diverse patient outcomes.

We prepared a list of clinical signs and symptoms, laboratory tests and imaging results related to different infectious pathologies. The ~120 cases included community- and healthcare-acquired pneumonia, viral and bacterial meningitis, urinary tract infection, influenza, cellulitis and *C. difficile* colitis, among others. The game provided players with clinical information about each patient gradually to help them decide the diagnosis and management for the case. Clinicians could opt to prescribe oral antibiotics, broad- or narrow-spectrum intravenous (IV) antibiotics, request further tests or discharge the patient without any treatment. In an attempt to replicate decision-making in real life, we developed a scoring algorithm that rewarded timely and accurate diagnosis and management and penalised rushed or delayed decisions. Delayed consequences of some prescribing choices were also made explicit to players using re-attending cases. For example, using IV antibiotics too frequently results in patients returning with cannula-site infections, thus increasing clinicians' workload. Likewise, the excessive use of broad-spectrum antibiotics will also lead to cases complaining of antibiotic-associated diarrhoea.

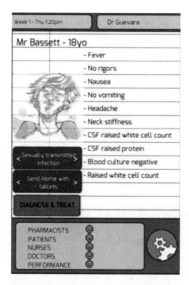

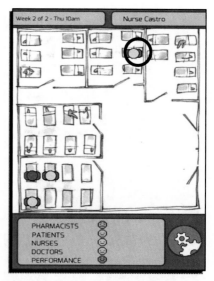

Fig. 1. Virtual patient with clinical symptoms and diagnosing options

Fig. 2. Gamification elements including timers, personalization, scores and multiple simultaneous cases

3.2 Gamification elements

Different features incorporated in the user interface promote constant interaction with the game. For example, personalization with players' name or the use of timers and scores encourage a continued engagement. The increasing case difficulty also contributes to sustained commitment to desired behaviours. Figure 2 illustrates the game mechanics and specific features included to focus players' mind on desired antimicrobial prescribing behaviours and to highlight unintended consequences.

Immediate feedback on performance is provided after each case and at key interim time points during the game (Figure 3). Such feedback fuses diagnostic accuracy and the impact of therapeutic decisions on other professionals and the wider hospital environment. Future versions of the game will allow players to print off their feedback and reports for inclusion in their professional portfolios; however, further work is required to generate evidence about the usefulness of this aspect of the game.

Additionally, behavioural nudges and messages are offered by peers and other professionals, patients, hospital management and governmental quality assurance inspectors, depending on each player's performance (Figure 4). Whilst these nudges have a humorous tone, they provide information about not only antimicrobial prescribing but also other associated patient safety behaviours such as hand hygiene or intravenous catheter use.

Other classic elements of gamification such as competition and social networking components could be incorporated in future iterations of the game. For example, individual players as well as clinical teams performance may be published (with their agreement) in a ranking, in addition to social networks.

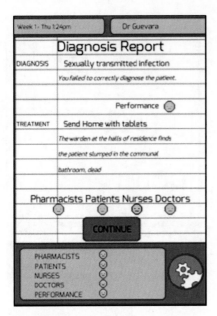
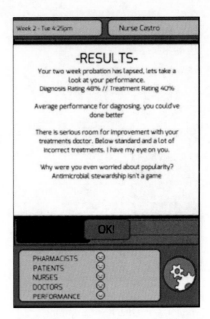

Fig. 3. Feedback following management of a case (left) and interim performance report (right)

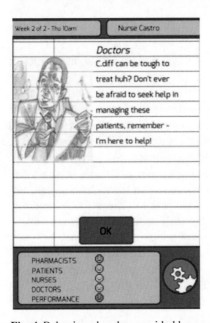

Fig. 4. Behavioural nudge provided by peer doctor

4   Evaluation

We propose to evaluate the game by combining qualitative and quantitative methodologies supplemented by in-game metrics.

4.1   Qualitative approaches

Players will be invited to participate in semi-structured interviews to explore their perceptions and opinions about using the game, and to discover whether they feel their practice may have changed. The qualitative, reflective methodology would also help identify any facilitating factors or barriers for engagement, as well as unintended effects. For example, a high level of playtime may reflect an elevated interest or an excellent response to the gamification elements included, but may, on the other hand, impact on the productivity of the participants.

4.2   Quantitative approaches

Two randomised controlled trials will provide information about the efficacy of the game. The first trial will be carried out amongst junior doctors starting their clinical rotations in our hospital organizations. The doctors recruited in this four-arm study will be randomised to receive either 1) a conventional educational session on antimicrobial prescribing, 2) a smartphone game unrelated to antimicrobial prescribing, 3) the serious antimicrobial prescribing game, or 4) the combination of educational session plus the serious antimicrobial prescribing game.

We will use vignettes with clinical scenarios to assess the knowledge, confidence and decision making of the participants on enrolment as well as at defined time points during the study period. Naturally, we would expect participants allocated to receive the educational package to obtain better results in the clinical vignettes requiring more or better knowledge of antimicrobials. However, participants using the prescribing game should, on the other hand, perform optimally in the behavioural vignettes.

The second trial will target 4th-year medical students and will utilise a modified version of the game to explore if those students randomised to receive the game achieve better scores in the end-of-year Prescribing Safety Assessment (PSA), a national exam jointly developed by the British Pharmacological Society and the Medical Schools Council to elicit competencies in relation to safe and effective use of medicines.

4.3   In-game metrics

Multiple parameters during gameplay are collected and transferred to an external database, using unique identifiers for each participant. From broader metrics such as engagement with the game or duration of each encounter, to the exact time required for participants to resolve each case and the diagnostic and therapeutic decisions made, or the influence of prompts and nudges on prescriber's decisions by the different characters (doctors, nurses, pharmacists, hospital managers) can be extracted and mapped. Potentially, we could identify favourable dose-effect relations i.e. whether increased gameplay time greatly improves prescribing decisions).

5   Discussion

Hitherto serious digital games in medical education, surgery and infection prevention and control have concentrated on providing technical knowledge or increasing manual dexterity. However, the ongoing initiative described here aims to influence prescribing behaviours amongst hospital doctors. The ubiquity of smartphone devices in our clinical setting, the increasing computing power of such devices, and the success of previous smartphone-based initiatives in our organization encouraged us to develop a serious antimicrobial prescribing game. Moreover, the psychological techniques and mechanisms frequently used in games, broadly identified as gamification, may resolve the difficulties associated with sustained engagement in behaviour change strategies.

The relative ease by which new cases can be added to the game engine allows for multiple possibilities. It would be possible to produce versions of the game tailored to particular clinical areas (i.e. immunodeficiency, paediatrics or tropical medicine), as well as settings with limited availability of antimicrobials. Furthermore, the game could be promptly modified to be useful in the learning of optimal behaviours in emerging infections such as Ebola.

6   Conclusions

Sustaining appropriate prescribing behaviours remains a challenge for antimicrobial stewardship actions worldwide. Serious games delivered on mobile devices can complement the experiential learning of prescribers. Games can be useful to reinforce desired behaviours, elicit the relationships between different professional groups involved in prescribing decision-making, and highlight any unintended consequences of antimicrobial prescribing. Serious games may be an affordable and feasible solution to address the behavioural and social influences on prescribing.

Acknowledgements: The research was funded by the National Institute for Health Research Health Protection Research Unit (NIHR HPRU) in Healthcare Associated Infection and Antimicrobial Resistance at Imperial College London in partnership with Public Health England (PHE). The views expressed are those of the author(s) and not necessarily those of the NHS, the NIHR, the Department of Health or Public Health England. The authors acknowledge the UKCRC who fund the Centre for Infection Prevention and Management at Imperial College London. Luke SP Moore and Myriam Gharbi acknowledge the support of the Imperial College Healthcare Trust NIHR Biomedical Research Centre (BRC).

7 References

[1] World Health Organization. Antimicrobial Resistance: No Action Today, No Cure Tomorrow. 2011.

[2] Dellit, T.H., Owens, R.C., McGowan, J.E. Jr, Gerding, D.N., Weinstein, R.A., Burke, J.P., Huskins, W.C., Paterson, D.L., Fishman, N.O., Carpenter, C.F., Brennan, P.J., Billeter, M., Hooton, T.M., Infectious Diseases Society of America, Society for Healthcare Epidemiology of America: Infectious Diseases Society of America and the Society for Healthcare Epidemiology of America guidelines for developing an institutional program to enhance antimicrobial stewardship. Clin.Infect.Dis. 15, 159-77 (2007)

[3] Charani, E., Castro-Sanchez, E., Sevdalis, N., et al. Understanding the determinants of antimicrobial prescribing within hospitals: the role of "prescribing etiquette". Clin. Infect. Dis. 57, 188-96 (2013)

[4] Jalink, M.B., Goris, J., Heineman, E., Pierie, J.P., ten Cate Hoedemaker, H.O: The effects of video games on laparoscopic simulator skills. Am. J. Surg. 208, 151-6 (2014)

[5] Kerfoot, B.P., Baker, H.: An online spaced-education game for global continuing medical education: a randomized trial. Ann. Surg. 256, 33-8 (2012). Erratum in: Ann. Surg. 256, 669 (2012)

[6] King, D., Greaves, F., Exeter, C., Darzi, A.: 'Gamification': influencing health behaviours with games. J. R. Soc. Med. 106, 76-8 (2013)

[7] Charani, E., Castro-Sánchez, E., Moore, L.S., Holmes, A.: Do smartphone applications in healthcare require a governance and legal framework? It depends on the application! BMC. Med. 14, 12-29 (2014)

Virtual Reality and *Mobius Floe*: Cognitive Distraction as Non-Pharmacological Analgesic for Pain Management

Amber Choo[1], Xin Tong[1], Diane Gromala[1] and Ari Hollander[2]

[1]School of Interactive Arts and Technology, Simon Fraser University, Surrey, B.C, Canada
{achoo, tongxint, dgromala}@sfu.ca
[2]Firsthand Technology Inc., Seattle, W.A, USA
ari@firsthand.com

Abstract. This paper outlines the intentions and current design behind the production of *Mobius Floe*, an immersive virtual reality game catered to acute and chronic pain patients. Researchers have shown that immersive virtual reality (VR) can serve as a non-pharmacological analgesic by inducing cognitive distraction in acute pain patients [Hoffman 2000]. *Mobius Floe* experiments with virtual reality as well as auditory immersion, a more experimental approach to cognitive distraction for pain relief; the results will be tested by acute as well as chronic pain patients to determine if chronic sufferers can benefit from similar VR practices as their acute counterparts. *Mobius Floe's* game design is informed by contemporary game design theory and cognitive psychology in order to improve its distractive properties.

Keywords. Chronic pain, acute pain, pain management, serious game design, health games, analgesia, virtual reality, cognitive load

1 Introduction

Virtual reality (VR) applications have yet to become a widely accepted complementary method to analgesics to reduce the perception of pain despite documented instances of its success. *SnowWorld*, a VR game with accompanying head mounted display (HMD) has demonstrated that VR treatments can work in tandem with pain medications to further reduce perceived instances of pain in patients with combat-related burn injuries [8]. Virtual reality has also been used to help combat other types of discomfort such as acute pain from dental procedures [6]. There is already evidence to suggest that chronic pain patients can benefit from immersive virtual reality applications [10]. Chronic pain patients, although requiring long-term pain reduction strategies, also suffer from shorter-term spikes in pain intensity [1] of which they may also benefit from non-pharmacological treatment practices suiting acute pain patients. *Mobius Floe*, the immersive VR discussed in this paper aims to expand upon non-pharmacological analgesic research for acute and chronic pain patients by improving the quality and variability of the distractive gameplay of its predecessors while introducing new forms of gameplay to examine, evaluate and compare to the field. Tasks involving cognitive distraction and heightened cognitive load are discussed for usage in *Mobius Floe* in order to attract and maintain the attention of pain patients.

2   Related Work

Virtual reality treatments for the reduction of acute pain have seen promising results in multiple studies. A VR titled *SnowWorld*, which draws patient's attention away from their embodied experience of pain and toward the virtual 3D environment was used to curb the wound care pain of U.S. soldiers injured with significant burns at the U.S. Army Institute of Surgical Research (USAISR). *SnowWorld* featured a snowy land-scape where the patient could throw snowballs and be hit by snowballs in the virtual space. This experience combined with analgesic medications served to improve the sol-dier's pain experiences in regards to "time spent thinking about pain" and experienced "pain unpleasantness", both of which declined significantly with the introduction of VR to their standard wound care routine [8].

Hoffman et al. reported significantly reduced levels of pain in dental patients under-going scaling and root planing in those who were immersed in cognitive distraction via a virtual reality simulation over patients who were asked to watch a movie and those who had no distraction present during their procedures [6]. Their results imply that immersive virtual reality applications may serve as an effective non-pharmacologic analgesic which could to be used in tandem with existing prescribed pain medications for dental pain; this conclusion by extension may also be applicable to other pain demo-graphics, especially considering the surrounding literature. For example, in a random-ized control trial study by Das et al., a virtual reality game was added to the proce-dural care schedule of children with acute burn injuries. The introduction of VR to their normally prescribed pharmacological analgesics decreased the average of the children's self-reported Faces Scale pain ratings from 4.1 (SD 2.9) to 1.3 (SD 1.8) [3].

The introduction of meaningful game design strategies can improve the gameplay of *Mobius Floe* to become more engaging than its previous counterparts, improving the quality of patient immersion. The examination of the potency of effects such as Csikszentmihalyi's 'flow' are important to maintaining virtual immersion, for flow "can be positively associated with degrees of the cognitive phenomenon of immersion and telepresence" [4]. *SnowWorld* has some degree of flow and is discussed widely in virtual reality literature. However, there is no perceivable consequence to inaction in *SnowWorld* when clear reactions from the game world in response to the player are necessary to create a more engaging design [2]. The *SnowWorld* patients also had minimal player agency in regards to their potential actions in the space, which is un-usual considering player agency is an extremely useful tool for user engagement [9]. *Mobius Floe* aims to learn from and improve upon previous attempts such as *Snow-World* by extending the software's ability to become immersive and cognitively dis-tract in a more reliable fashion.

Mobius Floe also incorporates techniques from the cognitive sciences by introducing n-back tasks, attentional switching and dual-task paradigms which work in tandem to invoke strong immersion, cognitive load, continuous action and heighten arousal

[5][11]. Patients are rewarded with 'health packs' to increase their player's health points (HP) when memorizing short visual patterns within the *Mobius Floe* space, recalling them later using a throwing mechanic to interact with the correct sequence of colors. Attentional switching and dual-task paradigm examples are discussed in the following section.

3 Virtual Reality Design and Development for *Mobius Floe*

Mobius Floe is currently being constructed in the Unity game engine and sports various distraction-based gameplay strategies in different areas of the virtual space. It can be played with the Oculus Rift head-mounted display (HMD) or a stereoscopic HMD provided by Firsthand Technologies, which sits in front of the eyes without touching the patient; the intent of using this hardware is to provide greater depth of cognitive immersion.

Mobius Floe appears as a sprawling snowy landscape, and the player is automatically moved forward through the space. The patient can look around the virtual space using the Oculus Rift or with a mouse as they are brought to their next destination.

The patient quickly finds themselves under threat from monsters which appear to be half neuron, half tree (see Fig. 1). These 'neuron trees' have menacing expressions and require sedation to escape from successfully. They chase the player and will damage their Health Points (HP) on contact. The neuron trees represent the neurological systems in the human body which are causing the pain experience; patients are able to calm them down by throwing abstracted particle systems representing analgesics with the left mouse button. The neuron trees serve as a key mode of cognitive distraction as they coerce the player into taking defensive actions against them in a strategic and time sensitive manner. Overuse of drugs against the neuron trees results in negative consequences, some of which manifest as detrimental behaviors in the neuron trees, while others affect the visual rendering of the virtual space in a negative fashion. For example,

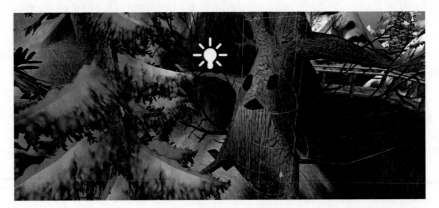

Fig. 1. A production still of *Mobius Floe* which shows an idling neuron tree.

overuse of morphine slows the neuron trees down considerably, but they become more aggressive once the effect wears off.

Sea otters also wander the virtual space and are able to interact with the patient (Fig. 2). They are friendly entities always approaching the player on sight, serving as metaphors for the patient's friends and family. Sea otters wag their tails and smile up at the patient when nearby. The patient can toss sea urchins at the otters in the same way they toss analgesics to the neuron trees. Otters who receive sea urchins will drop health packs for the player.

Occasionally the n-back tasks discussed in the previous section, sea otters and neuron trees will be in the proximity of the player at the same time, encouraging attentional switching and dual-task paradigms. The player must switch their attention between the neuron trees' location, the n-back task memorization, their health points, and the otters, fully engaging their cognitive load. For example, the player may find themselves fending off neuron trees, trying to memorize the n-back task hint and trying to feed the otters simultaneously.

4 Future Work

The retention of pain experience metaphors and how they translate to new patients would help distinguish *Mobius Floe* from ordinary games. For example, do the helpful sea otters naturally correlate to feelings of comfort, friends or family? How does the health point mechanic translate to patient's experiences? Do the depictions of drugs and how they operate in the virtual space realistically represent pain patient's affective experiences? We will conduct several case studies with patients from Greater Vancouver to help evaluate the existing pain experience metaphors as well as the effectiveness of cognitive distraction and perceived pain reduction within *Mobius Floe*. To do so will help situate the position of *Mobius Floe* within the research field and provide further context as to where the development of *Mobius Floe* should gravitate toward.

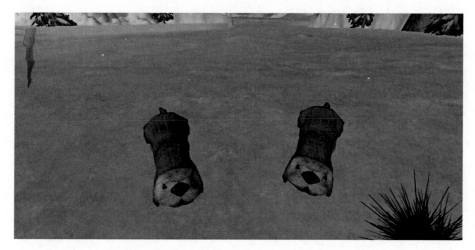

Fig. 2. Two otters greeting the player. 'HP' is visually represented as a red icicle in the top left.

5   References

[1] Baliki, Marwan et al. "Chronic Pain and the Emotional Brain: Specific Brain Activity Associated with Spontaneous Fluctuations of Intensity of Chronic Back Pain." The Journal of Neuroscience 26.47 (2006): 12165–12173.

[2] Church, Doug. "Formal Abstract Design Tools." Game Developer 6.8 (1999): 44.

[3] Das, Debashish et al. "The Efficacy of Playing a Virtual Reality Game in Modulating Pain for Children with Acute Burn Injuries: A Randomized Controlled Trial." BMC Pediatrics 5.1 (2005): n. pag.

[4] Faiola, Anthony et al. "Correlating the Effects of Flow and Telepresence in Virtual Worlds: Enhancing Our Understanding of User Behavior in Game-Based Learning." Computers in Human Behavior 29.3 (2003): 1113–1121.

[5] Herff, Christian et al. "Mental Workload during N-Back Task—quantified in the Prefrontal Cortex Using fNIRS." Frontiers in Human Neuroscience 7 (2013): 935.

[6] Hoffman, Hunter et al. "The Effectiveness of Virtual Reality for Dental Pain Control: A Case Study." Cyberpsychology & Behavior 4.4 (2001): 527–535.

[7] Hoffman, Hunter, David Patterson, and Gretchen Carrougher. "Use of Virtual Reality for Adjunctive Treatment of Adult Burn Pain During Physical Therapy: A Controlled Study." The Clinical Journal of Pain 16.3 (2000): 244–250.

[8] Maani, Christopher et al. "Pain Control During Wound Care for Combat-Related Burn Injuries Using Custom Articulated Arm Mounted Virtual Reality Goggles." Journal of CyberTherapy & Rehabilitation 1.2 (2008): 193–198.

[9] Schubert, Damion. "Narrative and Player Agency." Game Developer 18.2 (2011): 58.

[10] Shahrbanian, Shahnaz et al. "Scientific Evidence for the Effectiveness of Virtual Reality for Pain Reduction in Adults with Acute or Chronic Pain." 7 (2009): 40–43.

[11] Wickens, Christopher. "Multiple Resources and Performance Prediction." Theoretical Issues in Ergonomics Science 3.2 (2002): 159–177.

Gaming as a training tool to train cognitive skills in Emergency Medicine: how effective is it?

Mary E.W. Dankbaar[1], Maartje Bakhuys Roozeboom[2], Esther Oprins[2], Frans Rutten[3], Jan van Saase[1], Jeroen van Merrienboer[4] Stephanie C.E. Schuit[1,]

[1]Erasmus University Medical Center Rotterdam, the Netherlands.
[2]TNO, Soesterberg, the Netherlands.
[3]Training Institution for family practice, Utrecht, the Netherlands.
[4]Maastricht University, Institute for Education FHML, Maastricht, The Netherlands

Background and objectives

Training emergency care skills is critical for patient safety and an essential part of medical education. Increasing demands on competences of doctors and limited training budgets necessitate new and cost-effective training methods. In the last decade, serious games have been propagated to train complex skills; they are expected to facilitate active, engaging and intrinsically motivated learning. Erasmus MC has developed a serious game to train emergency care skills, as a preparation for the face-to-face training. This 'abcdeSIM' game provides a realistic online emergency department environment where doctors can assess and stabilize patients in a virtual emergency department.

Research questions: show residents, after using the abcde*SIM* game, better emergency care skills before f2f-training than residents who did not use the game? Are they feeling engaged with the patient cases and more motivated for the course?

Methods

In a quasi-experiment with residents preparing for a rotation in the emergency department, a 'nongame' group (n = 52) received a course manual and followed a 2-weeks certified f2f-training; the game group (n = 107) in addition received the *abcdeSIM* game before the same f2f-training. Emergency skills were assessed before training (in a subset of residents; n = 18 resp. n = 24) and at the end of the training, using a clinical and communication competency scale and an overall performance scale. Motivation and self-assessments were measured after the game with both groups; the game was evaluated using a questionnaire on engagement.

Results

After the game, before f2f-training, the game group performed better on clinical skills and the variety in scores was smaller compared to the nongame group (7-point scale; M = 4.3/3.5; SD = 0.75/1.27, p = .03; Cohen's d = .62). Scores on communication skills (M = 4.9/4.7, p = 0.52) and overall performance (M= 5.0/4.9, p= 0.93) were not different for both groups. Groups were comparable on main characteristics. At the end of the 2-weeks f2f-training, both groups performed similar on clinical skills (M = 5.7/5.6, p = 0.10). Results on the engagement questionnaire were positive (M= 3.9 on 5 pt. scale, 5 = very positive). Mean playing time was 2.2 hours, longer play was associated with higher game scores (r = 0.49, p < 0.001). Motivation for the course subjects (intrinsic value) for both groups was the same (7 pt scale; M = 6.2/6.1, p = 0.28 on).

Conclusions

After 2.2 hours spent playing a serious game on emergency skills, residents showed a substantial higher and more homogenous pre-training clinical skills level, compared to a comparable group who did not use the game. After 2 weeks training, there no longer was a measurable difference between groups. Serious games can be used as an effective preparatory training tool for complex skills. Further research will have to show whether f2f training can be shortened, maintaining the outcome level of training.

Games [4Therapy] Project:
Let'sTalk!

Menno Deen[1], Evelyn J.E. Heynen[2], Ben A.M. Schouten[3], Peer G.H.P van der Helm[4],
Andries M. Korebrits[2]

[1] Fontys ICT, Serious Gaming, Eindhoven, The Netherlands
menno.deen@fontys.nl
[2] Mondriaan, Heerlen, The Netherlands
(e.j.e.heynen, a.korebrits)mondriaan.nl
[3] Amsterdam University of Applied Sciences, Amsterdam, The Netherlands
ben.schouten@hva.nl
[4] University of Applied Sciences Leiden, Leiden, The Netherlands
helm.vd.p@hsleiden.nl

Abstract. 20% of Dutch youth suffer from psychiatric disorders that hamper their daily functioning and their personal development. Clients tend to drop out of school and have problems in their social environment. These clients often suffer from low social competencies and low empathic behavior, resulting in low treatment compliance. The study targets treatment motivation in order to prevent therapy dropout by introducing playful interventions.

Amongst others, social problem situations that arise from *interactions* between clients and their socio-cultural environment often lead to aggressive behavior and behavioral problems. It is not only the client, but also the reaction of the environment that plays an important part in the aggravation of clients' problems.

We focus on the group as a whole in order to gain insight these social interactions, to make them explicit and tangible, in an attempt to help clients (and their environment) to play and learn from these interactions, in order to contribute to a better social climate.

Keywords: serious game · mental health · empathy · e-health · motivation · therapy compliance · treatment motivation

Introduction

In the Netherlands, 20% of youth (aged 13 – 18) suffer from psychiatric disorders that hamper their daily functioning and their personal development [1]. There are other sources stating that approximately 225.000 young people could benefit from counseling [1]. Untreated, mental disorders can disrupt daily lives, cause social and economic loss and increase criminal behavior. Effective treatments can help restore well-being and executive functioning. Although many therapies have proven to be effective, a significant part of young adults appear difficult to treat [2, 3].

A common cause for treatment are inappropriate or aggressive reactions to social problem situations, low levels of empathy and low treatment motivation [4]. Results in aggressive behavior and high treatment drop-out [4, 5]. Treatment motivation has shown to be one of the basic features for successful treatment and rehabilitation [6]. Motivations is one aspect of treatment that appears highly relevant for progress and outcome of therapeutic interventions [7].

Within the domain of (mental) health, games and playful interventions have proven to be a successful communication tool for patients to express their feelings and problems without the need of verbal expressions . Research has shown that playful interventions can foster social negotiations [8]and may motivate players to engage in normally less desired activities [9]. Recently, applied games have found their way to train a small group of those clients. For example, clients with Attention Deficit/Hyperactivity Disorder (ADHD) are trained in planning their daily activities (*Plan-It Commander*) or executive functions (*Braingame Brian*) by playing Therapeutic Games.

Therapeutic Games can support clients outside their counseling sessions. Amongst others, they can train skills in within clients comfort zone, at home. *Braingame Brian* [10] has shown to improve executive functions. This proved to be effective for players' self-control [11, 12]. and is in line with studies on training executive functioning and it positive outcomes in clients with ADHD [13, 14].

At the moment of writing this paper, research is executed to validate influences of *Plan-It Commander* on planning skills and executive functioning amongst clients with ADHD. It is expected that playing the serious game can improve planning and communication in young children with ADHD. These games are single-player games and focus primarily on the client. Currently, there are no games or e-health applications that focus on the *interaction between clients and their social environment* [15].

This position paper of the *Games [4Therapy] Project* focuses on the interaction between children/adolescents and their relevant others in mental health care. These clients posses weak social competencies and show low empathic behavior. It is hard to engage this group in counseling. As a result, therapy-dropout is considerably high [16]. That is why we target treatment motivation in an attempt to decrease therapy dropout through the means of new digital forms of treatment.

Games or playful interventions may increase therapy compliance by boosting clients' motivation to stay engaged in therapy. Games have the ability to make abstract concepts concrete, tangible and playable and thus may help clients and their environment to create a better understanding of their problematic interactions. Also games can teach children to handle social problem situations (for example being disadvantaged, handling competition in a normal way and asking or giving help [5]. Enabling children to handle these social problem situations in a non-aggressive way will result in more positive feedback from peers and can contribute to a more positive social climate with their relevant others (transactional processes) [5].

Most interactions of youngsters take place during school time. That is why we will try to create a game that fosters positive social interactions amongst classmates with a central focus on clients' empathic behavior and social skills. The approach is to focus on the group as a whole in order to gain insight in the interactions, to make them explicit and tangible, with playful interaction and learning as a result.

Why Games and Playful Interventions?

Scholars and advocates from various disciplines already suggested that playful interventions can motivate players to engage in normally less attractive tasks. Games have shown to educate players implicitly about a rich variety of skills, like problem solving [17], strategic thinking [18] and leadership qualities [19]. This concerns implicit [18, 20, 21] as well as explicit learning [22, 23]. It is suggested that games can bring people closer together [24, 25], reduce pain during treatment [26, 27] or may even change the world for the better [28].

Most notably, games may positively effect players' motivation to engage in activities [29]. This appears especially true for games that offer players the opportunity to self-determine *how to play* [30]. Deen & Schouten [31] showed that students, who can experiment, explore and struggle with the learning content, reported to feel less controlled by their environment and to engage into learning practices after playing the game. They dubbed these games: autonomy-supportive. Autonomy supportive games present players with multiple solutions to a problem and offer them ways to play the game in the way they prefer.

We hypothesize that autonomy-supportive games or playful interventions may motivate clients to engage in therapy modules and tasks in their own way, and on their own time.

There are several reasons to choose playful interventions to motivate clients therapy engagement. Amongst others, games can offer a safe environment , create an emotional distance to the subject and/or problem , and can motivate clients to engage in activities they normally feel less inclined to engage in .

Safe Environment

Clients in therapy sessions often express anxiety and fear towards dealing with their mental issues[32]. It is therefore important that therapists create a safe environment in which clients can explore, experiment and struggle with their problems. Games can offer a kind of safe environment, mainly because making wrong decisions in games often does not have real life consequences. Juul [33] suggests that learning to cope with failure actually is one of the main advantages of playing and that it presents players with the most valuable learning opportunities. Juul's reasoning is best witnessed in so-called sandbox games [34, 35].

Sandbox games use its capacity to 'recruit diverse interests, creative problem solving, and productive acts' [36]. They create an environment for free and voluntary play that is called *Paidia* by Caillois [37]. These open games offer players the opportunity to change the rules and goals of the game [38, 39]. We consider this manipulation of the rules and regulations to be a playful activity, since play can essentially change, manipulate and rearrange existing structures to create something new [40] In short: a restructuring practice.

This restructuring can take place within the boundaries of a game. Often referred as the 'magic circle' [41, 42]. Derived from the works of Huizinga [43] the magic circle describes a liminal boundary that is in a constant state of flux and subject to social negotiations between players, designers and the rules themselves [8]. The boundaries of magic circle can create a safe environment in which it is clear, what is part of the game, and what not.

We hypothesize that games or playful interventions can offer a safe environment to play together with social relations by continuously negotiating about the boundaries of the game and the restructuring practices that take place.

Emotional Distance

The last reason to choose for a playful interaction is that gaming can create an emotional distance. We think that games can offer this emotional distance by making the client's problem explicit and tangible. This does create some challenges for designers. It may be hard to pinpoint which issues can be played and how one could transform a serious issues into an engaging activity.

Creating an emotional distance appears a natural way of coping [44]. Sometimes, when experiencing a socially problematic situation, friends suggest to consider the problem as a game. By doing so, someone can step back from one's own emotions, distancing themselves emotionally from feelings of hurt and anger, in an attempt to see what is happening. The emotional distance turns existing relations into tangible rules and into regulations that can be changed, or rearranged (BRON?). In short, viewing one own problems as a game may help people to play with social rules and regulations without being too emotionally involved.

It may seem odd to play with serious and real-life situations. However, game designers can make games out of everything: as Koven [25] states:

'We can play, [...] with everything – ideas, emotions, challenges, principles. We can play with fear, getting as close as possible to sheer terror, without ever being afraid. We can play with being other than we are – being famous, being mean, being a role, being a world.'

Making social relations explicit can help individuals to distance themselves from the emotional turmoil and ruminations that often follow a particular social problematic situation. Instead, the difficulties become tangible and playable. The difficulty from a designer's perspective is that this playful experience does not always have to be positive.

Play is by its nature an ambiguous concept [45]. It can be both, free and restricting, real and imagined, about you as about others. This offers a rich opportunity for designers and researchers to explore in the context of cognitive therapy.

We hypothesize that a game can present players with explicit and tangible relations that help them to take an emotional distance from their own and other's behavior, in order to facilitate constructive discussions about the problems that arise from the interactions between both parties.

Why Empathy and Motivation?

Currently, playful interventions, games and e-health applications appear to focus on training of cognitive activities and executive functioning in clients with mental health problems. The focus of those interventions is still on the problems of the client, whilst the reaction of the environment may influence the behavior of clients as well. Therefore, we focus on clients and their relevant others in the society.

Therapy programs for adolescents with mental health disorders follow a similar approach. These therapies place high emphasis on the interaction between clients and their environment. Although many therapies have proven to be effective in treating clients with low levels of empathy, a significant part of young adults appears difficult to treat [2, 3] and have a low treatment motivation [4].

Motivation describes the willingness of an individual to engage in an activity [46]. Amongst others, motivation is of significant importance to the effectiveness of psychic treatment. Low treatment motivation can result in high drop-out rates during treatment [5] especially in youngsters with externalizing problem behavior [4]. Treatment motivation has shown to be one of the basic features for successful treatment and rehabilitation and has been shown to be highly relevant for progress and outcome of therapeutic interventions [7].

Another common problem in adolescents with mental disorders is their failure to behave empathic towards others [47, 48]. Empathy is defined as, 'the tendency to apprehend another person's condition or state of mind' [49]. A failure in empathy can result in a failure to understand someone else's feelings, perspectives and behaviors.

Persons with low empathic competencies are less willing and able to regulate their emotions. They appear to suffer from impulsivity [50, 51], quickly resort to aggression, and they score low on fear conditioning [52]. Furthermore these clients have low impulse control, act and feel selfish, and can show psychopathic traits (for an overview see [50, 51, 53, 54]). Disorders like Schizophrenia, Psychopathy, antisocial personality disorders, depression and autism all deal with a low empathic behavior [48]. Targeting empathy may proof a fruitful approach to improve some issues that clients with externalizing problems deal with.

We hypothesize that games and playful interventions may be an interesting media to tackle social interactive problems and treatment motivation in youth. The Games [4Therapy] Project will investigate whether games can fosters pro-social behavior, empathy, treatment motivation and therapy compliance in adolescents with mental health disturbances.

Games For Therapy

The Games [4Therapy] Project focuses on children and adolescents in mental health care who have low social competencies and low empathic behavior, resulting in restricted treatment motivation. The study targets treatment motivation in order to prevent therapy dropout. The development of tools and interventions (games) outside (but part of) the counseling sessions may help those clients to keep engaged with their therapy in short moments over a prolonged timespan.

Therefore the expected study is looking into the next series of questions:

- How to improve (abstract and unclear) social relations or transactional processes between clients and their environment explicit and tangible, in order for clients to play with, and reflect on them?
- How to design a digital intervention that is not about training socially desired behavior or specific skills, but instead opens-up discussions and reflection upon the relationships between individuals? This way, we try to help groups to come-up with an effective solution that may improve their social climate, through a bottom-up approach.
- How to align the intervention with existing therapy? When should the interventions take place and who should be involved in the implementation and moderation of these social negotiations?

All these questions explore different design directions, in comparison with existing games for therapy. Whilst existing games focus on the client (only) and train specific skills and cognitive activities, we will focus on transactional processes in a group and facilitate conversations about socially problematic behavior in a playful way. We think that this may help clients and their relevant others to emotionally distance themselves from the problems at hand and discuss strategies to overcome. As a possible result, the distance may create a safe environment to express and reflect upon oneself, contributing to a better social climate.

In order to create a playful intervention we will align to the research by design approach [55, 56]. In this approach we start by creating low fidelity prototypes that are tested with the targeted audience and domain-experts. This will occur in early stages of the development, for the purpose of making valuable iterations on the interventions. The next 6 steps will explain our initial method to create an actual prototype of a playful intervention.

Step 1: Ethnographic Research

The game will be developed for boys and girls of Dutch special education secondary schools aged 12-18years who suffer from mental illnesses or learning disabilities. Desktop research, and non-scripted interviews with clients, peers and teachers will be utilized to get a better understanding of the social interactions that take place in this group.

Step 2: Connecting to Existing Therapies

After investigating and understanding the difficulties and possibilities of the social negotiations in classroom settings, a thorough study will be performed to existing therapies and their way of facilitating positive social interaction in the classrooms to create a better social climate.

Step 3: Game Jamming

The knowledge gained from above studies is disseminated to other game designers during a 'Game Jam' – an organized event to create playable prototypes in a very short time frame. 'Game Jams' offer a unique and quick way to prototype games. Beyond that, Game Jams can be seen as a design research method, situated in the research-through-design tradition, to create knowledge in a fast-paced, collaborative environment' [57]. The Games [4Health] Jam will present the research project with new insights, possible solutions and practical implications of our theoretical vision.

In May 2014 the first game jam was organized and it appeared rather difficult to transfer the knowledge of therapists to practical applications. Plenary sessions gave too little room for discussion between designers and domain experts. The premise to focus on social interaction did elicit interesting games in which players needed to communicate with each other in order to progress through the game. The study to co-operative multiplayer games turned out to be a worthwhile exercise. It shows how easy spatial path finding defuses the original intent of developers. The initial thought of some jammers was to elicit social negotiations. However, when the games progressed, jammers got distracted by the playful opportunities presenting itself during development. As a result the social negotiations related more to spatial orientation than to though issues. It appears that game jams with serious purposes would benefit from the inclusion of a domain expert during development sessions.

Step 4: Designing Ourselves

With the knowledge gained from the Games [4Health] Jam and the ethnographic study, games or playful interventions will be designed for therapy purposes. They will build upon personal experience or work close together with 'experience-experts' to create games.

For example, during the Lyst-Summit Game Jam in June 2014, game developers (Tim Pelgrim and Paul Bierhaus, YipYip; and Menno Deen, Lapp) worked together with a therapist for sexually abused children (Frank Lips, the Rading) and a victim of sexual abuse. Together the game *VilDu?* was created. The game is based on an existing therapy tool and targets issues that concern boundary setting. In the existing therapy tool, clients draw themselves on a big piece of paper. With color markers they depict whether and where they like to be touched. *VilDu?* enriches this activity with a social component, interactivity and the opportunity to limit someone else's actions.

VilDu? is a two-player game. It presents players with the opportunity to explore their natural curiosity to sex in a safe environment. In the game, players can perform various sexual actions by tapping and sliding over an iPad. Icons depict the acts of looking, touching, un-clothing, kissing, grabbing and licking. Players can unlock these acts step by step. If the other players does not appreciate a particular act, he/she can hit the stop button. The stop button clearly communicates the boundaries of the other player and locks the last unlocked sexual act on the other player's iPad.

VilDu? is a sexual exploration game for children that focuses upon depicting one's boundaries. It tries to communicate that sex is fun and that it is 'very ok' to set boundaries. From this design experience we learned how to communicate with therapists, which questions to ask during development and how a digital application could enrich existing therapy tools.

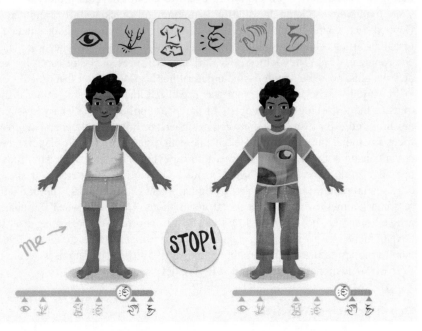

Fig. 1. *VilDu?* a game developed in 48 hour game jam during the Lyst-Summit 2014 in Copenhagen: it explores how an existing therapy tool can be enriched by digital means.

Step 5: Three Prototypes

After the prototyping and jam sessions, one of the most promising playful intervention will be developed into a prototype. From this prototype two/three different versions will be designed. The differences in designs will come from co-creation sessions with different experience experts (or end-users).

Step 6 User Testing & Validation

The final prototypes will be used in a classroom setting. To investigate the effects of the game on empathy, social interactions and treatment motivation there will be a pre-post test design. For example, *the Classroom Climate Inventory* [58], *the taxonomy of problematic social situation self-report* (TOPS) [4] and *the Basic empathy scale* [4] can be useful tools to investigate the effects of the expected games.

It is expected that the game elicits social negotiations about the behavior of both, clients and their significant others. These ´others´ are involved in the clients' developmental processes. Amongst others these are parents, teachers and friends. The expected playful intervention may improve social interactions and empathic behavior towards others, which may result in decreasing social problem situations and may improve treatment motivation due to an increased awareness of clients' personal problems and failures. Possibly the expected game/playful intervention will improve social competences and enhance treatment success.

Conclusion

Today, treatment procedures of adolescents with mental disorders are changing. Amongst others, financial needs for efficiency and innovations in (mental) e-health are responsible for this change. Budget cuts are commonplace in mental health institutions, and a strong governmental push to self-help can be witnessed in today's health systems. There appears to be a trend in which clients found their own health-foundations to accommodate their personal well-being. As a result, clients are becoming increasingly self-dependent.

In the Games [4Therapy] Project a multidimensional team of psychologists, game designers and researchers explore how to develop games as additional tools for therapies of different externalizing problem behaviors. It is hypothesized that the motivational aspects of games may contribute to a better engagement in normally less desired activities [28]. We will study how coping with social problem situations, emotional distancing, the creation of a safe environment, and the ability to play with social relationships may increase clients' therapy compliance.

Games have shown to increase engagement [59, 60] and overall motivation towards learning [9]. Many e-health interventions try to harness these motivational aspects of games and translate them to counseling or therapeutic tools. However, they mainly focus on the training of executive functioning and seem to be less concerned with the social environment and the social interactions that are taken place between clients and their significant others.

We examine the social interactions that take place between clients and their significant others to improve social interactions and their empathic understanding of others. Our goal is to create games/playful interventions that facilitate social negotiations between clients and their social environment, in an attempt to increase the empathic understanding of both groups, and contribute to a better social climate.

Acknowledgements. We would like to thank all the participants of the Games [4Health] Jam 2014 and all therapists involved in the event. In particular, we thank Frank Lips, Tim Pelgrim and Paul Bierhaus for their voluntary involvement in the Lys-Summit Game Jam, giving us the opportunity to experience the practical implications of our theoretical findings first hand.

References

[1]   1. Willems P, Rietveld J, Lahuis B, et al. (2011) Jeugd-ggz: Investeren in de toekomst! GGZ Nederland

[2] Lampropoulos GK (2011) Failure in psychotherapy: an introduction. J Clin Psychol 67:1093–1095.

[3] McKay D, Storch EA (2009) Cognitive-behavior therapy for children: treating complex and refractory cases. Springer Pub, New York

[4] Van der Helm GHP, Matthys W, Moonen X, et al. (2013) Measuring Inappropriate Responses of Adolescents to Problematic Social Situations in Secure Institutional and Correctional Youth Care: A Validation Study of the TOPS-A. J Interpers Violence 28:1579–1595.

[5] Edlund MJ, Wang PS, Berglund PA, et al. (2002) Dropping out of mental health treatment: patterns and predictors among epidemiological survey respondents in the United States and Ontario. Am J Psychiatry 159:845–851.

[6] Van der Helm GHP, Wissink IB, De Jongh T, Stams GJJM (2013) Measuring treatment motivation in secure juvenile facilities. Int J Offender Ther Comp Criminol 57:996–1008.

[7] Olver ME, Stockdale KC, Wormith JS (2011) A meta-analysis of predictors of offender treatment attrition and its relationship to recidivism. J Consult Clin Psychol 79:6–21.

[8] Copier M (2007) Beyond the magic circle: A network perspective on role-play in online games. Utrecht University

[9] Deen M, Schouten BAM (2011) Games that Motivate to Learn: Designing Serious Games by Identified Regulations. Handb. Res. Improv. Learn. Motiv. Educ. Games Multidiscip. Approaches

[10] Shosho (2010) Braingame Brian. PC

[11] Ten Brink E, Ponsioen A, Van der Oord S, Prins P (2011) Braingame brian. Kind Adolesc Prakt 10:166–174.

[12] Prins PJM, Ponsioen A, Ten Brink E (2011) Gebruik Je Hersens: Het verbeteren van executieve functies bij kinderen door oefening en training. Psycholoog 11:38–48.

[13] Klingberg T, Forssberg H, Westerberg H (2002) Increased Brain Activity in Frontal and Parietal Cortex Underlies the Development of Visuospatial Working Memory Capacity during Childhood. J Cogn Neurosci 14:1–10.

[14] Klingberg T, Fernell E, Olesen PJ, et al. (2005) Computerized training of working memory in children with ADHD-A randomized, controlled trial. J Am Acad Child Adolesc Psychiatry 44:177–186.

[15] Ruwaard J (2013) E-health in de jeugd-ggz – baat het of schaadt het?, v5 ed. Kenniscentrum Kinder- en Jeugdpsychiatrie, iTunes

[16] De Haan AM, Boon AE, de Jong JTVM, et al. (2013) A meta-analytic review on treatment dropout in child and adolescent outpatient mental health care. Clin Psychol Rev 33:698–711.

[17] Shaffer DW (2008) How Computer Games Help Children Learn. Palgrave Macmillan

[18] Gee J (2003) What Video Games Have to Teach Us About Learning and Literacy, 1st ed. Palgrave Macmillan

[19] Reeves B, Malone TW (2007) Leadership in Games and at Work: Implications for the Enterprise of Massively Multiplayer Online Role-playing Games. Seriosity

[20] Beck JC, Wade M (2004) Got Game: How a New Generation of Gamers Is Reshaping Business Forever, First Printing. Harvard Business School Press

[21] Johnson S (2005) Everything Bad Is Good for You: How Today's Popular Culture Is Actually Making Us Smarter, 1st ed. Riverhead Hardcover

[22] Aldrich C (2009) The Complete Guide to Simulations and Serious Games: How the Most Valuable Content Will be Created in the Age Beyond Gutenberg to Google. John Wiley & Sons

[23] Egenfeldt-Nielsen S (2005) Beyond Edutainment: Exploring the Educational Potential of Computer Games.

[24] Bekker T, Sturm J, Eggen B (2010) Designing playful interactions for social interaction and physical play. Pers Ubiquitous Comput 14:385–396.

[25] Koven BD (2013) The Well-Played Game: A Player's Philosophy. The MIT Press

[26] Van Twillert B, Bremer M, Faber AW (2007) Computer-Generated Virtual Reality to Control Pain and Anxiety in Pediatric and Adult Burn Patients During Wound Dressing Changes: J Burn Care Res 28:694–702.

[27] Hoffman HG, Patterson DR, Seibel E, et al. (2008) Virtual Reality Pain Control During Burn Wound Debridement in the Hydrotank: Clin J Pain 24:299–304.

[28] McGonigal J (2011) Reality Is Broken: Why Games Make Us Better and How They Can Change the World, 400th ed. Penguin Books

[29] Habgood MPJ, Ainsworth SE, Benford S (2005) Intrinsic Fantasy: Motivation and Affect in Educational Games Made by Children. Simul Gaming 36:483–498.

[30] Przybylski AK, Rigby CS, Ryan RM (2010) A Motivational Model of Video Game Engagement. Rev Gen Psychol 14:154–66.

[31] Deen M, Schouten BAM (inPress) The differences between Problem- Based and Drill & Practice games on motivations to learn.

[32] Breuk RE, Clauser C a. C, Stams GJJM, et al. (2007) The validity of questionnaire self-report of psychopathology and parent-child relationship quality in juvenile delinquents with psychiatric disorders. J Adolesc 30:761–771.

[33] Juul J (2013) The Art of Failure: An Essay on the Pain of Playing Video Games. The MIT Press

[34] Janssen C What is Sandbox? In: TechoPedia. http://www.techopedia.com/definition/3952/sandbox. Accessed 15 Apr 2013

[35] Weirdoloko J (2007) sandbox game. In: Urban Dict. http://www.urban-dictionary.com/define.php?term=sandbox%20game. Accessed 15 Apr 2013

[36] Squire K (2008) Open-ended video games: A model for developing learning for the interactive age. Open-End Video Games Model Dev Learn Interact Age 167–198.

[37] Caillois R (2001) Man, Play and Games, Reprint. University of Illinois Press

[38] DeKoven B (2004) Junkyard Sports, 1st ed. Human Kinetics

[39] Sihvonen T (2009) Players Unleashed!: ModdingThe Sims and the Culture of Gaming. University of Turku

[40] Deen M, Schouten BAM (2010) Let's Start Playing Games! how games can become more about playing and less about complying.

[41] Klabbers J (2006) The Magic Circle: Principles of Gaming & Simulation: Third and Revised Edition. Sense Publishers

[42] Salen K, Zimmerman E (2003) Rules of Play: Game Design Fundamentals. MIT Press

[43] Huizinga J (1951) Homo Ludens: Proeve Eener Bepaling van het Spel-Element der Cultuur. H.D. Tjeenk Willink & Zoon N.V., Haarlem

[44] Dyregrov A, Mitchell JT (1992) Work with traumatized children — Psychological effects and coping strategies. J Trauma Stress 5:5–17.

[45] Sutton-Smith B (1997) The Ambiguity of Play. Harvard University Press, Cambridge

[46] Ryan RM, Deci EL (2000) Self-determination theory and the facilitation of intrinsic motivation, social development, and well-being. Am Psychol 55:68–78.

[47] Jolliffe D, Farrington DP (2006) Development and validation of the Basic Empathy Scale. J Adolesc 29:589–611.

[48] Farrow TFD, Woodruff PWR (2007) Empathy in mental illness. Cambridge University Press, Cambridge; New York

[49] Johnson JA, Cheek JM, Smither R (1983) The structure of empathy. J Pers Soc Psychol 45:1299–1312.

[50] Davis MH (1994) Empathy: A social psychological approach. Westview Press, Boulder, CO, US

[51] Raine A (2013) The Anatomy of Violence: The Biological Roots of Crime. Random House LLC

[52] Popma A, Raine A (2006) Will future forensic assessment be neurobiologic? Child Adolesc Psychiatr Clin N Am 15:429–444, ix.

[53] Farrow/Woodruff Empathy in Mental Illness. Cambridge University Press

[54] Fairchild G, van Goozen SHM, Calder AJ, Goodyer IM (2013) Research Review: Evaluating and reformulating the developmental taxonomic theory of antisocial behaviour. J Child Psychol Psychiatry 54:924–940.

[55] Eladhari MP, Ollila EMI (2012) Design for Research Results: Experimental Prototyping and Play Testing. Simul Gaming 43:391–412.

[56] Laurel B (2004) Design Research: Methods and Perspectives. MIT Press

[57] Deen M, Cercos R, Chatman A, et al. (2014) Game jam: [4 research]. ACM Press, pp 25–28

[58] Van der Helm GHP, de Swart B, Stams GJJM (InPress) Back to school, measuring classroom climate in (semi) secure and prison schools.

[59] Habgood MPJ (2007) The effective integration of digital games and learning content. University of Nottingham

[60] Malone TW (1981) Toward a theory of intrinsically motivating instruction. Cogn Sci 5:333–369.

Tunnel Tail: A New Approach to Prevention

Mathea Falco[1], Jesse Schell[2], and Deidre Witan[3]

[1] Drug Strategies, Washington, D.C., United States
mathea.falco@gmail.com
[2] Carnegie Mellon University, Pittsburgh, Pennsylvania, United States
jesse@schellgames.com
[3] PB&Games, Somerville, Massachusetts, United States
deidre.witan@gmail.com

Abstract. This study determined the efficacy of the game *Tunnel Tail* in improving players' confidence in their ability to resist illegal drugs and alcohol. 246 students in the target age group of 11 to 13 years old were given a survey before and after playing *Tunnel Tail*. Players were split into two groups, which played either one or two twenty-minute sessions. Session length was based on data of average play time. Comparing survey responses before and after gameplay, 86% of active players showed improvement in at least one area of resistance attitudes. Players who reported reading and paying attention to the in-game dialogue showed greater improvement. Additionally, longer play time was correlated with increased confidence in resistance behaviors. Despite its limitations (small sample, lack of control group), the survey suggests that a larger study is warranted. Tunnel Tail provides an early glimpse of the potential for using sophisticated game apps to enhance learning of resistance skills and effect behavior change.

Keywords: adolescent substance abuse prevention, resistance skills, efficacy survey, mobile game app, drug use prevention

1   Introduction

Adolescent smoking, drinking, and drug use remain a major concern in the United States. The most recent National Survey on Drug Use and Health estimated that 2.4 million children ages 12-17 were current drug users, meaning that they had used illicit drugs in the past month before the survey [1]. Experimentation with substances begins early in life: among 8th graders, 19% reported having tried an illicit drug in 2012, while 15% reported having used tobacco and 30% had drunk alcohol [2].

In order for drug prevention efforts to be effective, they must target youth at the age at which they begin experimenting with substances [3]. This is important in light of the fact that the research shows that the earlier young people start to use substances, the more likely they are to experience adverse outcomes [4]. For the past three decades, school-based drug education curricula, supported by billions of dollars in federal government funding, have been the primary approach to prevention. However, many of these programs have not been rigorously evaluated, and those that have often fail to show overall reductions in drug use. Moreover, effects of even the best programs fade unless booster sessions are provided in high school [5]. At the same time, schools have come under increasing pressure from academic testing requirements, and severe budget cuts have reduced teaching staff and classroom hours. As a result, drug prevention in most public schools has largely disappeared or been reduced to a few sessions in middle school. New approaches to drug education and prevention are urgently needed.

Tunnel Tail is a major innovation in the prevention field: a highly engaging, complex mobile game built on important prevention concepts and designed to reach adolescents ages 11-13 outside the classroom by bringing prevention messages directly to them on their mobile devices, where they spend much of their time.

The primary purpose of this survey was to determine if the game was effective in changing attitudes surrounding drug use, specifically players' confidence in resisting pressure to use drugs and their motivation to do so. If Tunnel Tail shows positive effects in improving resistance skills among young adolescent players, it could point the way to a new generation of sophisticated prevention game apps to enhance learning of resistance skills and possibly effect behavior change.

2   Methods

Tunnel Tail, an award-winning free game app built on key prevention concepts, is designed to reach youth where they spend many of their waking hours: communicating and playing games on hand-held devices [6]. Developed for the BEST Foundation by Schell Games in consultation with Drug Strategies, Tunnel Tail targets adolescents 11-13 years old, when they begin experimenting with alcohol, tobacco and drugs [3]. Early focus testing found that this age group reacts very negatively to direct reference to anything resembling formal "drug education." Consequently, the game mechanics and dialogue use metaphors that build on key prevention concepts embedded in the text and game play, rather than on more direct didactic formats that often characterize traditional classroom-based prevention curricula. Specifically, the game is designed to introduce players to situations where they may feel pressures to use substances and how to deal with those situations, to show that players don't need to give in to pressures to be cool, to engage players in positive peer support, and to provide different scenarios for trying out resistance skills. Players practice those resistance skills through repetitive game play that encourages incidental learning as they advance through the game. While the design and conceptual framework of the game app is built on key findings of prevention research of the past two decades, [7,8] Tunnel Tail takes an entirely new approach to prevention messaging.

Tunnel Tail is a sophisticated role-playing game with complex graphics and player interactions built for iPhone and Android platforms. The main characters are intelligent mice who live with humans in real world settings and must confront the Controllers, who are trying to take over their world. The mice, despite their size, can become powerful when they stand up for themselves, take control of the situation and help other mice. The core element of the combat system is the pressure mechanic that displays different levels of pressure depending on the scenario and provides different methods for players to respond. Players level up with each effective response to pressure situations. Through its multiplayer features, the game emphasizes relationships, leadership, confidence and learning to take control. Although playing through the entire game takes about ten hours, most kids play intermittently; they may leave the game for several weeks and then return. Everything is saved, so they can continue playing where they left off.

Extensive focus group testing with the target adolescent age group influenced the graphics, design and game play. Engaging both girls and boys was an important priority. For example, the game uses turn-based play, rather than aim-and -shoot fights, because they proved to be popular with both boys and girls. Players can also customize their mice with different outfits and equipment, an option especially attractive to girls, while the toughness of the mouse characters appealed particularly to boys.

Tunnel Tail was launched as a free app in September, 2012; by June, 2013, there had been 255,000 downloads. Of this group, 40 percent are active players. Tunnel Tail is highly rated both on Google Play (4.2 stars) and iTunes (4 stars). The app was a finalist at the 2012 Serious Games Challenge, runner-up for overall best digital game at Meaningful Play 2012, and won a Silver Medal at the 2013 International Serious Play Award.

3 Design

This study employed a two group pre-post design. Participants were randomly assigned to the two groups. Respondents were divided into segments based on gameplay assignment and gender:

- Short-Play Respondents (n=109): played Tunnel Tail once for 20 minutes.
- Long-Play Respondents (n=137): played Tunnel Tail twice for 20 minutes each, with a break of at least 4 hours in between.
- Males (n=155)
- Females (n=91)

A set of questions addressing the game's appeal, memorable aspects, and core messages was given before and after gameplay to assess changes in answers between pre- and post-gameplay.

4 Participants

246 male and female gamers, ages 11 to 13, participated in the study. Within the target audience, all respondents regularly played other games on mobile devices (iOS/Android phones or tablets). VGMarket, a market research firm specializing in the videogame industry, conducted an online survey in May 2013. Using online and phone screening, 246 eligible subjects were recruited from VGMarket's database of over 250,000 video game players. (Funding limitations for the study capped the number of participants at 250.) Subjects were screened for age, gender distribution, and familiarity with other mobile games. Because the survey was conducted online, subjects were located in at least 18 different states, however, 30.5% did not disclose their

address. Informed verbal consent was obtained both from parents of the adolescents and the adolescents who participated in the online survey. The questions were developed at the Harvard Graduate School of Education's Technology, Innovation and Education Program in consultation with Drug Strategies.

5   Procedures

Players were divided into a "short-play" group (20 minutes) and a "long play" group (two 20 minute sessions separated by at least four hours). This format of 1 or 2 20-minute sessions was based on the average gameplay time, based on the statistics provided by Schell Games. According to their metrics, 72.1% of active players play at least 2 battles, which is easily achieved within the first 20 minutes of the game. This means that the results from the short-play group are directly applicable to at least 72.1% of active players. Additionally, 28.4% of active players obtain a second mouse, which occurs after about 40 minutes of total gameplay. By testing players at 20 and 40 minutes, we were able to get a good assessment of the majority of players. Furthermore, Schell Games designed Tunnel Tail to be played casually in short spurts, so having the long-play group log out of the online survey between their 20-minute play sessions fit with the overall design for the game.

6   Data Analysis

6.1   Comparison of Pre- and Post-Gameplay Questions

Players were asked similar questions before and after gameplay about their perceived abilities to recognize and resist peer pressure. The vast majority of players exhibited changes in their answers between these pre- and post-gameplay questions. These changes did not all reflect an improvement in peer resistance confidence and attitudes, but 86% of the respondents did exhibit at least one positive (reflecting improvement) change in their responses after playing the game.

In addition, players were asked what they were paying attention to and what they remembered after they had finished playing. There was a statistically significant correlation between players who indicated that they did remember the dialogue and those who exhibited positive changes between pre- and post-gameplay answers ($P< 0.001$).

Additionally, students who reported reading the in-game dialogue also exhibited a significantly higher number of positive changes ($P=0.043$). Conversely, there was also a correlation between the students who indicated that they did not read the in-game dialogue and the number of negative changes they exhibited in pre- and post-gameplay questions ($P =0.035$). This indicates that the in-game dialogue is crucial to the game's success as a prevention tool.

6.2   Comparison of Short- and Long-play Groups

Longer play time was significantly correlated with a higher confidence in ability to leave a situation where drugs and/or alcohol are being used. One question measured players' confidence in their abilities to avoid and refuse illegal drugs by asking for their confidence level on five different resistance behaviors. There was a statistically significant correlation between play time length and the level of confidence in their ability to leave a pressuring situation ($P=0.025$).

Additionally, a higher percentage of players identified a key message of the game in the long-play group. The percent of players who identified *If you practice standing up for yourself, your skills will improve* as a core message of the game increased from 70.6% of the short-play group to 81% of the long-play group. This is strong evidence of the positive effects of increased gameplay time ($P=0.057$).

6.3   Evidence of Appeal

When asked, "Would you keep playing the game past the point where you were asked to stop?" 33.7% of students reported that they "definitely would" continue playing the game, which was a higher percentage than any other answer. Among boys, 39% of those in the long-play group reported that they "definitely would" continue playing the game, as opposed to 23% in the short-play group. There was a statistically significant correlation between players' answers to this question and whether or not they read the in-game dialogue ($P<0.001$), however, it is unclear if reading the dialogue helped players enjoy the game more, or if enjoyment of the game helped players remember the dialogue.

In addition, 77% of the students would have chosen to play for longer than their allotted time. 80% of the long-play group, as compared to 73% of the short-play group, reported that they would like to continue playing, which indicates strong replay value.

When asked to what words accurately describe the game, only 4% chose "educational." The most popular responses were "interesting" (59%), "fun" (47%), and "addictive (34%).[1] There was a statistically significant correlation between the long-play group and those who characterized the game as "educational" ($P = 0.026$), which indicates that the longer a player is exposed to the game, the more likely they are to see the intentional educational messages.

7   Discussion

Tunnel Tail's purpose was to model resistance strategies in order to help players identify pressuring situations and practice healthy responses. The evidence suggests that playing Tunnel Tail helped students practice resistance skills as well as increase their confidence in their abilities to resist peer pressure to use drugs. A majority of players showed improvement between pre- and post-gameplay questions, and those improvements were correlated with reading and remembering the in-game dialogue. In addition, longer game play was significantly correlated with higher confidence in a players' ability to leave a situation where drugs and/or alcohol are being used.

The implications of these results are limited by the survey's small sample size, the lack of a control group, and the limitations of attempting to measure true behavior

---

[1]   Respondents could choose more than one answer

change through a written survey. In addition, the fact that both negative and positive changes in answer choices between pre- and post-gameplay questions were exhibited lowers the significance of any inferences that can be made.

Table 1. Survey and Responses

Before Gameplay:

How much do you agree/disagree with these statements?	Completely agree	Mostly agree	Mostly disagree	Completely disagree
I am very social and like meeting new people	46%	43%	9%	3%
I can't always tell when someone is trying to manipulate me	5%	28%	48%	20%
I have no idea what to say when a friend disagrees with me	3%	11%	53%	33%
I often think things through and plan ahead	28%	53%	17%	2%
I often let other people get their way to avoid a conflict	3%	37%	43%	16%
I often play multiplayer video games	43%	37%	15%	4%
Doing what I want is more important to me than fitting in	24%	56%	16%	4%
I can easily express my emotions	30%	51%	17%	2%
I stand up for myself when my friends and I disagree	37%	55%	7%	1%
Sometimes I need time to be alone	31%	50%	12%	7%
It's not important for friends to like the same things	18%	52%	24%	5%
I will do something I think is too risky if my friends encourage me	3%	17%	47%	33%

After gameplay:

	Definitely	31%
	Probably would	26%
Would you keep playing the game past the point where you were asked to stop?	Maybe would	20%
	Probably wouldn't	13%
	Definitely wouldn't	3%
	I would have stopped earlier	8%

	Interesting	59%
	Fun	47%
What words accurately describe this game? (Choose all that apply)	Addictive	34%
	Exciting	30%
	Boring	30%
	Hard	13%
	Educational	4%

	No fun at all	14%
	It was fun, but most other games are more fun	24%
	More fun than a *few* other games	17%
Compared to other free mobile phone games you've played, how much fun was Tunnel Tail?	About as much fun as other games	16%
	More fun than a *lot* of other games	17%
	More fun than most other games	9%
	The most fun mobile game I've played	3%

	It helped me understand what was going on	52%
	I enjoyed finding out more about the story	36%
	Too many dialogue screens	28%
	I got impatient to get to the next mission or battle	28%
The mice sometimes talk to you and each other outside of battle. What did you think? (Choose as many as apply)[2]	I often clicked through the screens without reading them	28%
	It helped me get to know the characters	26%
	I would have liked to learn more about the characters and story	20%
	Too much text on each screen	17%
	I don't remember what the mice said	16%

---

[2]   Included pictures of the referenced aspects of the game

During battle, the mice make comments to each other. What were the most memorable comments? (Does not have to be exact)[2]	Respondents filled in a text box with their answers

What are some ways that the ideas in Tunnel Tail can address real-life problems?	Expressed in the game (% Yes)	Helpful in real life (% Yes)	% Yes to both
Mice sometimes fight with each other	93%	27%	n/a
It's easier to stand firm when you have the support of your friends	74%	93%	69%
Working hard now will lead to rewards later on	76%	93%	n/a
It's best to stick to your own territory	54%	43%	n/a
Paying attention to the tension level helps in conflict	89%	69%	63%
Better equipment makes it easier to win	85%	61%	n/a
If you practice standing up for yourself, your skills will improve	80%	92%	76%
Sometimes enemies will say nice things to try win you over	90%	79%	73%
You should treat others the way you'd like to be treated	48%	93%	n/a

Thanks so much for giving us feedback on Tunnel Tail! The following questions will now ask you about your thoughts on issues outside of the game.

A friend of yours is pushing you to do something you don't want to. How likely are you to respond in each of these ways?	Definitely would	Probably would	Maybe would	Probably wouldn't	Definitely wouldn't
Give it a try – you might enjoy it	4%	17%	41%	18%	20%
Do what he wants to do now, and then do something you like later	6%	17%	27%	27%	22%
Provide an alternate suggestion	22%	45%	27%	4%	3%
Say that maybe you'll do it later	6%	23%	34%	19%	18%
Change the subject to talk about something else	15%	36%	31%	12%	7%
Make fun of her for wanting to do it	1%	6%	9%	32%	53%
Firmly say no and stick to it	30%	26%	29%	11%	4%
Get a friend to back you up	11%	30%	39%	14%	7%
Walk away	12%	22%	26%	24%	16%

How much do you think people risk harming themselves (physically and in other ways) if they…	No risk	Moderate risk	Great risk
Smoke one or more packs of cigarettes a day	2%	8%	90%
Skip class	14%	50%	36%
Ride in a car	42%	54%	4%
Ride in a car without wearing a seat belt	4%	38%	58%
Try an illegal drug once	3%	28%	69%
Regularly use illegal drugs	3%	4%	93%
Fly in an airplane	42%	52%	6%
Parachute out of an airplane	7%	53%	40%
Get drunk	4%	24%	72%
Ride a motorcycle without a helmet	2%	21%	77%

People differ in whether or not they disapprove of people doing certain things. How much do you disapprove of people doing each of the following?	Approve	Disapprove	Strongly disapprove
Smoke one or more packs of cigarettes a day	2%	13%	85%
Skip class	6%	46%	48%
Ride in a car	95%	3%	2%
Ride in a car without wearing a seat belt	5%	46%	49%
Try an illegal drug once	4%	24%	73%
Regularly use illegal drugs	2%	6%	92%
Fly in an airplane	90%	5%	4%
Parachute out of an airplane	49%	37%	14%
Get drunk	5%	26%	68%
Ride a motorcycle without a helmet	5%	26%	69%

How sure are you on each of these questions?	Not at all sure	Moderately unsure	Moderately sure	Completely sure
Can you refuse an offer of alcohol or illegal drugs?	2%	2%	13%	84%
Can you think of a way to stop someone who is pressuring you to drink or do drugs without making them angry?	3%	9%	48%	40%
Can you avoid situations where you know other people will be drinking or doing drugs?	2%	6%	27%	65%
Can you think of a way to leave a party where people are drinking or using drugs - without being made fun of?	2%	8%	31%	59%

Can you say "no" in a serious way and stick to it when a friend is pressuring you to drink or use drugs?	1%	3%	20%	76%

How much do you agree/disagree with these statements?	Completely agree	Mostly agree	Mostly disagree	Completely disagree
I know what to say when a friend disagrees with me	32%	50%	13%	4%
I don't always stand up for myself when my friends and I disagree	6%	18%	43%	33%
It's important for friends to like the same things	7%	37%	36%	20%
I won't do something I think is too risky even if my friends encourage me	46%	39%	11%	4%
I don't let other people get their way to avoid a conflict	16%	40%	35%	9%
Fitting in is more important to me than doing what I want to do	3%	12%	48%	37%
I can always tell when someone is trying to manipulate me	31%	49%	15%	5%

Table 2. Short- and Long-Play Group Procedures

Short-Play Group	Long-Play Group
Pre-gameplay question	Pre-Gameplay question
One 20-minute play session	One 20-minute play session
Immediately take survey	Wait at least 4 hours (no activities specified for this period)
	Second 20-minute play session
Survey Questions 1-10	Survey Questions 1-10
Post-gameplay question	Post-gameplay question

Table 3. Answers to the question, "Can you think of a way to leave a party where people are drinking or using drugs - without being made fun of?[3]

	Short Play	Long Play
Completely sure	49.54%	66.42%
Moderately sure	37.61%	26.28%
Moderately unsure	12.84%	7.30%

[3] The response of "completely unsure" has been omitted from this table for clarity, as no respondent chose that answer.

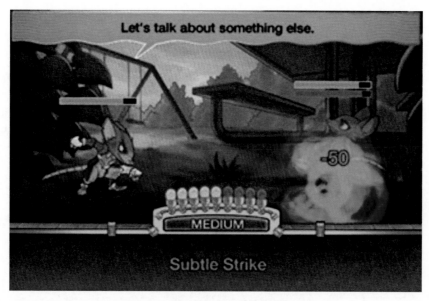

Fig. 1. Screen Capture from Tunnel Tail

References

[1] Substance Abuse and Mental Health Services Administration. Results from the 2012 National Survey on Drug Use and Health: Summary of National Findings, NSDUH Series H-46, HHS Publication No. (SMA) 13-4795. Rockville (MD): Substance Abuse and Mental Health Services Administration (2013) http://www.samhsa.gov/data/NSDUH/2012SummNatFindDetTables/National Findings/NSDUHresults2012.htm

[2] Johnston L., O'Malley P., Bachman J., Schulenberg J.: Monitoring the Future, National Survey Results on Drug Use, 1975-2012: Volume 1, Secondary School Students. Ann Arbor (MI): University of Michigan Institute for Social Research (2012) http://www.monitoringthefuture.org/pubs/monographs/mtf-vol1_2012.pdf

[3] The National Center on Addiction and Substance Abuse at Columbia University. Adolescent substance use: America's #1 public health problem. New York: Columbia University (2011) http://www.casacolumbia.org/upload/2011/20110629adolescentsubstanceuse.pdf

[4] Merline A, O'Malley P, Schulenberg J, et al.: Substance use among adults 35 years of age: Prevalence, adulthood predictors, and impact of adolescent substance use. Am J Public Health 94, 96-102 (2004)

[5] Botvin G., Griffin K.: School-based programmes to prevent alcohol, tobacco and other drug use. Int Rev Psych 19(6), 607-615 (2007)

[6] Common Sense Media. Do smart phones = smart kids? The impact of the mobile explosion on America's kids, families, and schools. San Francisco (CA):

Common Sense Media; (2010) http://www.itu.int/council/groups/wg-cop/second-meeting-june-2010/CommonSenseSmartPhonesSmartKidsWhitePaper.pdf

[7] Botvin G., Baker E., Dusenbury L., Botvin E., Diaz T.: Long-term Follow-up Results of a Randomized Drug Abuse Prevention Trial in a White Middle-class Population. JAMA. 273, 1106-1112 (1995)

[8] Spoth R., Redmond C., Trudeau L., Shin CR., et al.: Longitudinal Substance Initiation Outcomes for a Universal Preventive Intervention Combining Family and School Programs. Psychology of Addictive Behavior. 16, 129-134 (2002)

Game Design of a Health Game for Supporting the Compliance of Adolescents with Diabetes

Regina Friess, Nina Kolas, Johannes Knoch

Hochschule Furtwangen University, Fakultät Digitale Medien,
Robert-Gerwig-Platz 1, 78120 Furtwangen
regina.friess@hs-furtwangen.de, nina.kolas@hs-furtwangen.de,
johannes.knoch@hs-furtwangen.de

Abstract. Diabetes heavily impacts the day-to-day routine of those affected and requires a large degree of self-control and discipline. Since the disease is incurable, patients must learn to self-identify with their situation. In the case of adolescents, the basic problem of diabetes patients is exacerbated by several aspects. They are under high social pressure to conform with the expectations and want to be recognized in the group. They often find themselves in spontaneous situations and expose themselves more than adults to extreme physical experiences. They no longer simply submit to instructions from parents, guardians, or other adults. These factors result in adolescent diabetics being exposed to the danger of taking their medication incorrectly or inadequately, which consequently entails far-reaching risks to their health.

An approach to prevent this problem may be offered by a Serious Game, which is developed specifically for this need. The main objective of the game would be to promote the compliance of the affected person with diabetes treatment. It is meant to raise the awareness of the adolescents regarding the need to accept the disease and to face life with the sense of responsibility that the situation requires.

A conceptual prototype of a Serious Game is to be developed, which will make it possible for adolescent diabetics to identify better with their situation and to take more responsibility for their physical health. The paper presents a human-centred design process in the field of Serious Games.

Keywords: serious game, game design, compliance, adolescents, diabetes, stealth learning

1   Requirements and Project Goals

As an actual report about diabetes in Germany, it is a disease that is increasing rapidly in our society, especially for children and young adults. Diabetes is one of the most frequently occurring chronic diseases and metabolic disease in these age-groups (Danner 2014). A doubling of the rate of Type 1 diabetes for under 5-year aged is expected for the next six years. Moreover, Type 2 diabetes is also heavily increasing. During the last ten years the rate of juvenile-onset diabetic has multiplied by five (Danner 2014).

As Fink et al. (2014) state in their report on the social dimensions of diabetes, mellitus families with diabetic children are under a severe pressure. There is only little knowledge about the disease in public and the children are very often discriminated. Teachers find themselves overcharged in observing diabetic children during the different situations of school activities and deny taking responsibility for their health. (Fink et al. 2014). There is only minimal support from the public and from health institutions for the families.

Based on expert interviews with the psychologists Dr. Isolde Krug and Dr. Michael Barth of the Center for Pediatrics of the Medial Center – University of Freiburg[1] we extracted the following depiction of the problems that juvenile diabetics find themselves confronted with.

Diabetes requires a constant awareness and anticipatory planning during everyday life, which is contradictory to spontaneous activities and the often extreme experiences juveniles undertake. As they want to be accepted amongst their peer group, they often feel pressured to hide or ignore the conspicuous actions of medicating themselves. In addition, juveniles are much more than capable than adults to compensate the physical effects of a hypo-glycemic or hyper-glycemic state and therefore risk ignoring even more serious life-threatening conditions. Adolescent diabetics no longer simply submit to instructions from parents, guardians, or other adults in the way younger diabetics do. These factors result in adolescent diabetics who are more likely than other age groups to take their medication incorrectly or inadequately, which exposes them to far-reaching health risks.

An approach to prevent this problem may be offered by a *Serious Game,* which can be developed specifically for this need. As stated by the Psychologists, there is no need for the target group for further education on the necessity and the handling of the medical treatment, just as it would be more counterproductive then helpful to point out the potential risks of a disregardful handling of the disease. According to their professional knowledge, the aim must be to support the adolescents in finding a positive way of taking care of their health and to accept their exceptional condition.

Therefore, the main objective of the game would be to promote the compliance of the affected person with appropriate diabetes treatment. It is meant to raise the awareness of the adolescents in regards to the need of accepting the disease and to face life with the necessary responsibility that the situation requires.

2   First Approach for Game Concept

The preceding conceptual decisions give only a rough concept, which should be enhanced and evaluated in further research work. They are founded on the one hand on pragmatic restrictions (a 3D-Roleplaygame would exceed the capacities of the given team and the monetary resources) and on the other hand they match the central demands we extracted from the first expert interviews with the psychologists. The

---

[1]   Interviews took place in March 2014 and were conducted by a project group of Prof. Dr. Regina Friess, within the Master Design of Interactive Media at University of Furtwangen.

central aspects we wanted to cover with the game concept were: Refer to the constant additional task-layer diabetics have to fulfil; give a heroic image to persons who have to manage this task and show that they therefore have to build up special forces; refer to the positive aspects of a social backing.

The game will be developed on the basis of a simple and well-known game genre (Jump and Run). The particular demands of diabetic adolescents will be addressed using metaphorical transferred game situations. The central approach is the parallelism of simultaneous demands and objectives in different situations to which the protagonists see themselves as being exposed in real life. The basic game mechanic of the genre will be altered by adding a second autonomic task layer concerning the vitality of the main character. Thereby the player will have to manage a double tasking role throughout the whole game. This will metaphorically address the additional burden that the diabetic adolescents have to sustain in everyday live.

The narrative part will focus on the main character, who is a sympathetic hero with a handicap, which gives him/her the aura of being special but not perfect. Because of this it is important to have a good friend. There will be a sidekick that assists during adventures that the protagonists will undertake. The representation of the world and the actions will be designed as a two dimensional comic. Because of his/her special physical disability which is very difficult to keep balanced throughout the game, the hero will experience flashy visions or exceptional skills according to his or her different states in life. These effects might either be positive or negative with regard to the overall game objectives.

3 Theoretical foundation

The theoretical approach refers to an understanding of media perception based on concepts of symbolic interaction. It postulates a sociological perspective on meaning construction in digital culture and mediated communication aiming on a procedural analysis going beyond concepts of motivation and gratification (Krotz 1996). Processes of meaning construction are analysed as activities related to social concepts of the self and others, the pragmatic situations framing the constructive processes, and the interdependence between media perception and social interaction with, for example, friends and peer groups (Krotz 1996).

As Claudia Wegener highlights, the process of media acquirement has become a central concept within this sociological perspectives on media usage. It is assumed that media structures everyday lives, especially of younger generations and in multiple ways (Wegener 2007).

Shared media experiences can help to reflect and foster the discussion of real problems or relevant issues, either alone or with others and in several ways (Krotz 1996).[2]

---

[2] Andreas Hepp (1999) discusses the relevance of communicative patterns, which establish an intersubjective process of relating media experiences to the everyday context.

On one hand, personal issues can be discussed on a substitutional basis, referring to fictional agents and representative situations. As these characters are fictional, people can even discuss intimate issues without being offended or feeling ashamed.[3]

On the other hand, representations of social situations or structures in fictional narration and game settings are always reductive. Narrative structures are selective and help to build causal relations (Branigan 1998). Game structures establish a selective set of dependencies and build systematic relations (Frasca 2003). In both ways they reduce real live situations and can help to handle the complexity.

It is assumed that in games, narrative and playful forms of meaningful construction and user involvement take place (Friess 2012). The narrative concept helps to get involved with agents situated in an ongoing action. Main components are motivations and intentions in relation to assumed conflicts or objectives[4] (Smith 1995). According to Grodal (2007) narrative patterns help us to anticipate possible situations and build emotional hierarchies on an imaginative level: how would I evaluate this situation and how would I decide? Grodal opposes two general directions of narrative coping of situations – either change an undesirable state (taking action) or find a way to accept an unchangeable situation (Grodal 2007). The second option would lead either to a melodramatic narration or by trying to cope with the unchangeable by taking distance through comical or ironical representations (Grodal 2007). In our case the situation is unchangeable and the task is to find a way of accepting it. Therefore, a comic distance could be helpful to convey a less depressing perspective on one´s fate. A similar effect of cathartic relief can be achieved through the possibility of transgressive behaviour within the protected bounds of game play (Sutton-Smith 1972) which unburdens the player, for example, from physical constraints and social pressure of real live situations.

Playful involvement is determined by a task-oriented involvement referring to the player himself and his capability of managing different situations (Grodal 2000). Main components are interesting tasks, an affordance of action, perceived possibilities, and the allowance for experimental exploration. A balanced relationship between the perceived affordance and an assumed capability of being successful in fulfilling the tasks fosters a constant involvement (Klimmt 2003). Suspense is given by the unpredictability of upcoming situations and outcomes of one's own actions as well as the uncertainty of one´s own capability of coping with these tasks. (Grodal 2007). These components are central for a successful game involvement and must be part of the conceptual evaluation.

It is assumed that the playful component of meaning construction focusses more on structural understanding of interdependencies (Frasca 2003) in order to be able to manipulate the given system in a projected manner. Therefore an intended reference to experiences in everyday live in a serious game should focus on a simulative adap-

---

[3] See the considerations of Angela Keppler (1995) to the topic of identification with fictional characters in series. In her argument the figurative simplification of the characters even simplify and enhance the possibilities to refer to them in everyday communication and support a playful identification.

[4] This refers to an action oriented narrative setting, differing from a narration with a focus on situational description or mental processes (Lämmert 1955)

tion of action-oriented structures (Zimmermann 2010). As Witting showed in a qualitative research on processes of transference between real world and game play, there can be transfers of several categories (e.g. action patterns or mental structures) and in both directions from real live to game play and vice versa (Witting 2007). We assume that in our case the structural similarities mainly based on the principle of constant double taxation will allow for recognition of everyday structures on one hand and may encourage a positive transfer to coping strategies in real live on the other hand.

4   Data collection by expert interviews as basic for concept of the serious game

In this research project a social scientific study is integrated in order to explore how the development of a serious game enables young diabetics to identify with their situation and to resume a higher responsibility for their health. The *available resources* are, among supervising doctors and psychologists, between five and seven young diabetics who will be consulted during the process of the game design. Later they will evaluate it as well.

The persons who are questioned in this project will be interviewed *personally*. The qualitative interview is still believed to be the standard instrument of empiric social research for the investigation of knowledge, opinions, attitudes or estimations in the social scientific scope (Phillips 1971, Kaase et al. 1983; Schnell et al. 2005).

The interview situation with the young diabetics will be partially structured (Atteslander 1984) because these are well suited for interviewing single persons. As an instrument of a qualitative social research, the benefit of a guideline based interview is that, because of the open conversation techniques and the expansion of answer margins, the scope of the respondent can be captured by the reply. In this way, we can gain the respondents structures of relevance and backgrounds of experiences (Schnell et al. 2005).

The subjects for the interviews on the first appointment with the partners for the study are:

1. Social demographics
2. Illness experiences (start of illness, physical experiences and symptomatology, reflection of illness, behavior with illness, everyday life, difficulties)
3. Social milieu (in most different connections to diabetes, behavior, difficulties)
4. Personal interests
5. Media usage (generally, Games, Computer Games)
6. Personal ideas about computer games and estimations of design proposals (character, p.r.n. "sidekick" included, settings, game situations, basic mechanics)

The results should highlight the typical difficulties concerning the illness – may these be difficulties in everyday life or problems because of the disease that are based on social milieu (1., 2. and 3.). The part concerning terms of media (4., 5. and 6.) should show the connection of the interview partners to media and to computer games, and it should show first design preferences of the diabetics. Those will be specified with several follow up interviews. The amount of all basic information, the score and the analysis of all interviews result in the basic of concept and the realization of the serious game.

However, before the accomplishment of the expert talks, a pretest will be conducted which should eliminate potential deficiencies of the inquiry. The pretest is focused on

- checking questions on comprehensiveness
- as good as possible investigation variances of answers which are expected
- investigating potential difficulties which interview partners can have on answering the questions
- checking the theoretical validity of the interview (Häder 2006).

The young diabetics will be involved with the development process of the serious game. A step by step development of the character, which the persons can identify themselves with, should be specified by several guided interviews; they will have a basic influence on the characters visual design and his/her temperamental direction. In the same way will be generated metaphorically from everyday life the diabetic's adapted settings, game situations, and game mechanics – focused on preferably meaningful adaptations of main difficulties from the group of the aforementioned mentioned subjects 2 and 3.

The next step is the *analysis* of previously transliterated qualitative interviews, and therefore, an orientation should be the analysis procedure of Mayring (1993), who structures it into three steps:

- Summary: basic testimonies of the text will be summarized and reduced to single categories.
- Explication: meaning analysis of "problematic" seeming passages – using other materials/sources is recommended.
- Structuring: structure attributes of the text will be filtered out by using a category system.

There should be both proposals of character design, of settings, of game situations, basic mechanics (from the first expert interviews), and the result – the finished prototype of the serious game. This result is to be evaluated by the interview partners. The proposal of designs (for example of the main character) and its evaluation is a very subjective undertaking, meaning they should merely be indicatory. Because of this reason the proposals will be evaluated by the respondents only roughly, for example, the *visualizing of the main character*: Is the character more likeable or more unlikeable? Why? What attributes are positive and what are negative? What is very appealing and what is not? Evaluations are specific advice for enforcing people; the efficiency of the approach must be proven in further detail. Expectations neither of enforcing people nor of the evaluating people are allowed to influence the findings of the evaluation project (Häder 2006).

5 Conceptual approaches

5.1 Methodology of Game Development

Nielsen (1963) showed that involving the target group during the design process is more efficient and effective than at the ending. By conceptualising several alternatives, the designers can get through an evaluation feedback and improve the concepts. This will reduce misinterpretations in the testing phase at a non-iterative process. This kind of exploratory process retrieves the target group and their needs, which can then be implemented directly (Nielsen 1993).

"In serious gaming projects, again in general, there is a minimum of three stakeholders: the designer, the deployer, and the player or client" (Wartena et al. 2014). In this project, the players are adolescents with diabetes, the designer and deployer are the students of the Hochschule Furtwangen University. A fourth role takes over the psychologists, who give input for a better understanding of the adolescents as well as for the conceptual approaches. However, an essential role has the adolescents, who are also the game designer. They will be involved during the entire process: (1) requirements engineering, (2) concept, (3) design, (4) prototyping and (5) evaluation as referring to the Rational Unified Process (RUP) (Kruchten 2004). Because of this sensible issue and the target group, we prefer to use human-centred activities to focus on the users, their needs and requirements (ISO 9241-210:2010) in order to achieve good results. There must be a repetitive cycle of design and evaluation (Gould et al. 1985), and this will be structured as followed:

1. Requirements engineering: First of all the psychologists and medical caregivers of adolescent diabetics at the university hospital in Freiburg serve as the basis for this *Serious Game*. According to an expert interview a set of issues could be surveyed and served as basis for the first approach for a game concept.
2. Concept: In a second interview with the adolescents, three different conceptual approaches of games are introduced. Three different main characters and sidekicks – in three different styles – stories, and game worlds are to be scribbled. These small concepts are evaluated and preferences of the gaming concepts given. In the interviews, there are also asked questions about their life and media usage behaviour. With these results, the design of the serious game can be continued.
3. Design: In the design phase the refinement of the characters, game world, mechanic and story will be developed. Because of the iterative, human-centred process, the target group will be questioned once more. The feedback will be analysed and inwrought in the design. This phase will start in October 2014.
4. Prototyping: After the design phase, an initial interactive mock-up can be implemented.
5. Evaluation: The playable characters, game world, mechanic and story will be evaluated. If the results are satisfying, the game will be developed according to the given feedback.

The first results from the interviews showed that the game should not refer too directly to structures of the disease, as this would lower the fun experience. This endorses the decision to refer to central aspects of the disease´s impact on everyday live on a metaphorical level.[5]

The main problems we detected were more or less confirmed with an additional aspect: even if you do behave very correctly, there is always the possibility of some surprise effects as the components of the physical condition, especially for adolescents, and the impact of the disease are too complex to be completely projectable.

5.2 Early concept prototypes

As described in chapter 2 the game will be based in the Jump and Run genre, which will also include action-elements. The protagonist in the 2D game will be a hero with a handicap, who has to fulfil tasks that may get him/her into a tangle or further into mortal danger. Based on the diabetes disease, the protagonist has to achieve balance during the entire game. It is a simplified metaphor for measuring the blood sugar level. A further metaphor is the sidekick, which represents the social environment. That serves to help the protagonist in difficult situations which he/she cannot handle alone.

In the current game development process, three different conceptual approaches were initiated:

- A neutral fantasy character which is situated in a magical world by accident. Because of the magical legacy, the character now has to control its power and achieve balance in life. With the help of its hat (which is also the sidekick), the protagonist can handle the situation.
- The protagonist is a hybridization of an animal and robot and lives in a steam-punk-/sci-fi-like world. During an explosion, the balance of its energy was damaged. The hybrid and its supportive butler (sidekick) have to save the world from ruin.
- The anti-hero is a fence in Havana, who was anaesthetised by his boss. He removed his pancreas and from now on has to handle his blood sugar level. At the beginning of the game, he meets the daughter of his boss (sidekick), who helps the protagonist during the game.

All three conceptual approaches have three basic elements: the protagonist with handicap, a supportive sidekick, and a so-called sugar meter.

Due to the indirect mapping on reality, the game should have a change process with regards to identification, awareness, acceptance and motivation, as well as positive effects to the compliance.

---

[5] Therefore the core concept differs from approaches, which represent the aspects of the medical treatment of diabetes, as for e.g. the Project GRIP. (see: http://www.ranj.com/content/werk/grip#.U9TjIUjTO6Y, 26.06.2014) This project focuses on the self-esteem of the affected adolescents and the social aspects of the disease.

6 Future Work

This project is a work in progress. After the evaluation of the interviews with the adolescents with diabetes, the elaboration phase and analysis and design discipline of the Rational Unified Process can be continued. According to the interviews with the adolescents, the preferred concept will be finalized, regarding the characters (protagonist and sidekick), story, and game world. After the design phase, the adolescents will be interviewed again. This feedback will be integrated as well. In the last phase, a prototype will be implemented and evaluated by the same target group. If the results are positive, the prototype can be developed.

7 References

[1] Atteslander, P. (1984): Methoden der empirischen Sozialforschung. 5. Auflage, Berlin: de Gruyter GmbH & Co. KG.

[2] Branigan, Edward (1998): Narrative Comprehension and Film. London, New York: Routledge.

[3] Danner, Thomas; Ziegler, Ralph (2014): Diabetes bei Kindern und Jugendlichen. In: Deutsche Dieabetes-Hilfe (ed.). Deutscher Gesundheitsbericht Diabetes 2014, Verlag Kirchheim + Co GmbH, Mainz 2014, pp. 126-135.

[4] diabetesDE – Deutsche Diabetes-Hilfe (Hg.) (2014): Deutscher Gesundheitsbericht Diabetes 2014. Mainz: Kirchheim + Co GmbH.

[5] Finck, Hermann; Holl, Reinhard; Ebert, Oliver (2014): Die soziale Dimension des Diabetes mellitus. In: Deutsche Diabetes-Hilfe (ed.). Deutscher Gesundheitsbericht Diabetes 2014, Verlag Kirchheim + Co GmbH, Mainz 2014, pp. 146-156.

[6] Frasca, Gonzalo (2003): Simulation versus Narrative: Introduction to Ludology: In: Wolf, Mark J. P.;Perron, Bernard: The Video Game Theory Reader. New York: Routledge, pp. 221-236.

[7] Friess;Regina (2012): Symbolic Interaction in Digital Games: Theoretical Reflections on Dimension of Meaning Construction in Digital Gameplay: In (eds.): Fromme, Johannes; Unger, Alexander: Computer Games and New Media Cultures: A Handbook on Digital Game Studies. Springer Verlag, Dordrecht u.a., pp. 249-264

[8] Gould, John D.; Lewis, Clayton (1985): Designing for usability: key principles and what designers think. In: *Commun. ACM* 28 (3), S. 300–311. DOI: 10.1145/3166.3170.

[9] Grodal, Torben (2000): Video Games and the Pleasure of Control: In: Zillmann, Dolf; Vorderer, Peter (Hrsg.). Media Entertainment: The Psychology of Its Appeal. Mahwah, London: S. 197-213.

[10] Häder, M. (2006): Empirische Sozialforschung – Eine Einführung. Wiesbaden: VS Verlag für Sozialforschung.

[11] Hepp, Andreas (1999): Das Lokale trifft das Globale: Fernsehaneignung als Vermittlungsprozess zwischen Medien- und Alltagsdiskussion. In: Hepp, And-

reas; Winter, Rainer (eds.): Kultur – Medien – Macht: Cultural Studies und Medienanalyse. Opladen: Westdeutscher Verlag, pp. 191-211.

[12] Holl, Reinhard W.; Grabert, Matthias (2014): Versorgung von Kindern und Jugendlichen mit Diabetes – Entwicklungen der letzten 18 Jahre. In: diabetes-DE – Deutsche Diabetes-Hilfe (Hg.): Deutscher Gesundheitsbericht Diabetes 2014. Mainz: Kirchheim + Co GmbH, S. 136–145.

[13] ISO 9241-210:2010 210, 03.03.2010: Ergonomics of human-system interaction — Part 210: Human-centred design for interactive systems. Online verfügbar unter https://www.iso.org/obp/ui/#iso:std:iso:9241:-210:ed-1:v1:en, zuletzt geprüft am 22.04.2014.

[14] Kaase, M./Ott, W./Scheuch E.K. (Hrsg.) (1983): Empirische Sozialforschung in der modernen Gesellschaft. Frankfurt am Main: Campus.

[15] Keppler, Angela (1995): Person und Figur. Identifikationsangebote im Fernsehen. In: Montage a/v, 4/2, pp. 85-99.

[16] Klimmt, Christoph (2003): Dimensions and Determinants of the Enjoyment of Playing Digital Games: . In: Copier, Marinka;Raessens, Joost: Level Up: Digital Games Reserach Conference. Utrecht: Utrecht University, S. 246-257.

[17] Krotz, Friedrich (1996): Der symbolisch-interaktionistische Beitrag zur Untersuchung von Mediennutzung und -rezeption. In: Hasebrink, Uwe; Krotz, Friedrich (eds.). Die Zuschauer als Fernsehregisseure? Zum Verständnis individueller Nutzungs- und Rezeptionsmuster, pp. 52-75. Nomos, Baden-Baden/ Hamburg.

[18] Kruchten, Philippe (2004): The rational unified process. An introduction. 3. ed. Boston [etc.]: Addison-Wesley (The Addison-Wesley object technology series).

[19] Lämmert, Eberhard (1955): Bauformen des Erzählens. . Stuttgart: Metzler.

[20] Mayring, P. (1993): Qualitative Inhaltsanalyse. Grundlagen und Techniken. 4. Auflage, Weinheim: Deutscher Studienverlag.

[21] Nielsen, Jakob (1993): Iterative user-interface design. In: *Computer* (11), S. 32–41. DOI: 10.1109/2.241424.

[22] Schnell, R./Hill, P. B./Esser, E. (2013): Methoden der empirischen Sozialforschung. 10. Auflage, München: Oldenbourg Wissenschaftsverlag GmbH.

[23] Schouten, Ben; Fedtke, Stephen; Bekker, Tilde; Schijven, Marlies (Hg.): Games for health. Proceedings of the 3rd conference on gaming and playful interaction in health care.

[24] Smith, Murray (1995): Engaging Characters. Fiction, Emotion and the Cinema. Oxford: Clarendon Press.

[25] Sutton-Smith, Brian (1972): Die Dialektik des Spiels. Schorndorf: Karl Hofmann Verlag.

[26] Wartena, Bard O.; Dijk, Hylke W.: Bias Blaster – Aiding Cognitive Bias Modification- Interpretation through a bubble shooter induced gameflow. In: Ben Schouten, Stephen Fedtke, Tilde Bekker und Marlies Schijven (Hg.): Games for health. Proceedings of the 3rd conference on gaming and playful interaction in health care, S. 47–60, zuletzt geprüft am 25.04.2014.

[27] Wegener, Claudia (2007). Stichwort: Medienforschung in der Erziehungs-wissenschaft. In: Zeitschrift für Erziehungswissenschaft, December 2007, Volume 10, Issue 4, pp 459-477.

[28] Witting, Tanja (2007): Wie Computerspiele uns beeinflussen. Transferprozes-se beim Bildschirmspiel im Erleben der User. München: Kopaed.

[29] Zimmerman, Eric (2010). Learning to play to learn. http://www.ericzimmerman.com/texts/learningtoplay.html, (25.04.2014)

The Effect of Social Sharing Games and Game Performance on Motivation to Play Brain Games

Jeana H. Frost[1,*], Allison L. Eden[1]

[1] VU University Amsterdam
{j.h.frost,a.l.eden}@vu.nl

Abstract. Brain games can be an effective way to help people "train" and maintain cognitive agility over time. Although game content is based on well-established tasks, the means to motivate people to play remains more of an art than a science. This paper tests the impact of different types of feedback commonly used in entertainment-oriented games on intrinsic motivation, enjoyment and performance within a brain game. In a 2 by 2 factorial design, we compare performance-based feedback (a score) with task completion feedback (a badge) and two contexts for that feedback, private (viewed independently) versus shared (posted on a social network). Shared feedback is associated with higher motivation and game enjoyment. There is no difference in level of performance on intrinsic motivation. Contrast analysis and pairwise comparisons reveal that the shared and performance-based feedback is most motivating. We discuss the implications for brain games specifically and interventions more broadly.

Keywords: motivation, feedback, gamification, brain games, social media.

1   Introduction

Within the lab setting, psychologists use well-established tasks to test and "train" particular cognitive abilities, including attention and working memory in order to preserve function. Although performing these tasks regularly may have long-term benefits for cognition, [1, 2, 3] it can be difficult to motivate people to do mental exercises now in order to improve cognitive health in the distant future. One way to transform even the simplest, routine task into something fun is through "gamification," adding game elements and attractive interface design to otherwise repetitive tasks [4, 5]. If well designed, the resulting activities, labeled "brain games," may be just as engaging as other simple, short games people play purely for entertainment. Although the design of brain games is based on psychology research, with the contents of the game consisting of well-understood laboratory tasks [3], the best methods to motivate users to play these games remains more of an art than a science. However, designers of brain games can learn from game design and research in other domains. Game designers routinely use and study mechanisms such as feedback and posting and sharing game experiences through social networks in order to heighten the appeal of game play. In this study, we test the use of these mechanisms within brain games.

Although game feedback, e.g. badges and points, are central to the design of a game, research suggests that feedback can have either constructive or deleterious effects on game enjoyment and motivation depending on its form and interpretation [6, 7]. In this study, we empirically test two types of feedback: performance based (points) and completion based (badges).

In addition, while brain games are becoming more popular, game play remains largely an individual-level experience with users playing on their own. Yet, the popularity of playing games and posting activity on online social networks suggests that social sharing can improve the game experience and perhaps heighten motivation.

Based on the rise in popularity of Social Network Games (SNGs), and informed by theory on human motivation, the current study compares the use of privately viewed game feedback to socially shared feedback on intrinsic motivation, enjoyment and performance within a brain game.

2 Theory

2.1 Motivation

There are two types of motivation: first, intrinsic motivation, which refers to the inherent satisfaction associated with performing an activity; second, extrinsic motivation, which is contingent on a external reward (e.g. monetary compensation)[8]. In the case of brain games, while they are designed to raise long-term cognitive health, this extrinsic reward rarely occurs immediately. The benefits are long-term and difficult for an individual to perceive. Therefore, the current study focuses on intrinsic motivation and more immediate payoffs, such as game enjoyment.

2.2 Feedback and Motivation

When people play SNGs, they receive scores and badges as a result of game play. The effect of feedback on intrinsic motivation is hotly debated. According to Deci, Koestner and Ryan [6], the effects of feedback are contingent. Feedback can either help people feel more competent, thereby raising intrinsic motivation, or be perceived as reducing autonomy, thereby suppressing intrinsic motivation. Cameron and Pierce argue that in applied settings, feedback mechanisms heighten intrinsic motivation, particularly for dull tasks [7]. This debate suggests that the characteristics and interpretation of feedback matter for motivation and the use of feedback to raise motivation would benefit from further study.

2.3 The Social Environment and Shared Feedback

Despite a wealth of work on feedback, there is surprisingly little literature on how the social environment affects intrinsic motivation. The closest studies examine the effect of verbal encouragement on intrinsic motivation. Deci, Koestner, & Ryan [6] suggest that, as for other types of feedback, the value of verbal encouragement depends upon how that feedback is interpreted. If feedback from others is perceived as controlling, then it is damaging to intrinsic motivation; if feedback from others is understood as a source of information, then it increases intrinsic motivation [9].

One possible mechanism linking socially shared feedback to motivation and behavioral change is that social sharing triggers social comparison [10], which in turn leads to heightened motivation. Social comparisons—competition in particular—heighten game enjoyment, which can be used as a proxy for intrinsic motivation [11]. While people play SNGs either by themselves or asynchronously, they may still feel competitive with others in the knowledge that outcomes are socially shared. As a related example, although people do not necessarily play arcade games with others, leader boards post previous "high scores" to implicitly promote comparisons among gamers, enticing them to perform better and attain higher scores.

2.4 Structuring the Feedback

How feedback is structured within games may contribute to both the level of social comparisons players make and the intrinsic motivation they experience. According to the reward classification model suggested by Wang and Sun, players perceive the highest level of social comparison and competition when feedback is both public and marks progress in game performance. Although there are a variety of feedback formats, Wang and Sun state that game score, the simplest display of task performance, is one of the best ways to elicit social comparisons; it is easy to understand and communicate. Scores may be motivating because, in contrast to displays of task completion, such as a badge, they reflect a level of competence within the game, which leads to greater intrinsic motivation [8].

Building upon past research, we will look at two feedback structures: first, private versus socially shared feedback, and second, task completion versus performance-based feedback, assessing how these impact intrinsic motivation, enjoyment, interest, and perceived competition in a simulated brain game. We predict that public, performance-based feedback will increase enjoyment, interest, and perceived competition of the game, which will lead to increased motivation to play.

3 Method and Procedure

3.1 Participants

We recruited a total of 202 people (88 men, 114 women, Mage = 25.6, SDage = 8.04, 97% Dutch) through online advertisements posted on social network sites such as Facebook and Twitter. 99 per cent of participants had Facebook profiles, 64 per cent LinkedIn, 46 per cent Twitter, 29.7 per cent Instagram, 20 per cent Hyves, 7.5 per cent Foursquare, 3 per cent MySpace, and 5 per cent indicated they were members of other social network sites such as Pinterest, Tumblr, Google+, and QQ. An analysis of the distribution of responses revealed a normal distribution of responses across all types of social media use. Participants report a mean of 0.40 hours (SD = .80) spent on playing online games and a mean of 0.31 hours (SD = .75) playing network games daily.

3.2   Game and Procedure

We used a two factorial design. Participants were randomly assigned to either task or performance-based feedback (a badge or a score), either private or social feedback (shown to themselves or told it would appear on a study Facebook page), resulting in four conditions: social badge (N = 51), social score (N = 50), private badge (N = 51), private score (N= 50). After reading an introductory message, participants were told how they would receive their feedback and viewed a screenshot of that display. See figure 1.

Subjects then read the instructions and played a "brain game" resembling an existing game designed by neurologists to test attention (Neuroimaging, 2013). In the game, players closely watch a series of quickly flashing images that include two images from a specific category (e.g. two types of dogs) and then, after viewing the series of images, select which one (e.g. which picture of a dog) appeared second in the display. Players played ten rounds, gaining one point each time they correctly identified the second image.

After finishing the game, the respondents filled in items on motivation to play again, enjoyment of the game, and how competitive they found the game. Finally, respondents answered questions about demographics and current social media use. After finishing the survey, participants were debriefed and thanked for their time.

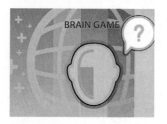 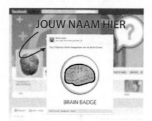 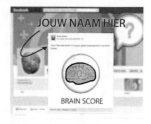

| A.   Private Conditions | B.   Social Badge | C.   Social Score |

Fig. 1. In the introduction, subjects previewed how their feedback would be displayed either privately, as a badge or score (A), as a badge on Facebook (B) or as a score on Facebook (C).

3.3   Measures

Intrinsic motivation. We measured motivation with two questions on a 7 point agreement scale anchored at 1 = 'No, totally not' and 7 = 'Yes, very much', phrased as 'Do you want to continue playing, after finishing this questionnaire?' and 'Do you wish to play this game another time?' The items together formed a composite scale, M = 3.70, SD = 1.53, Cronbach's alpha = .85).

Enjoyment. To measure enjoyment, we modified an existing questionnaire by (Teo, Lim, & Lai, 1999) measuring enjoyment along eight dimensions. A principal components analysis of these items revealed two distinct factors: Enjoyment (Frustrating-Fun, Unpleasant-Pleasant, Negative-Positive; M = 4.93, SD = 1.00, Cronbach's alpha = .84) and Interest (Dull-Challenging, Stupid-Intelligent, Boring-Exciting, Disinteresting-Interesting, M = 4.64, SD = .91, Cronbach's alpha = .81).

Competition. To measure if the respondents perceived this game as competitive, we asked one question: 'Do you perceive this game as competitive?' (7-point scale 1 = 'Totally not competitive' and 7 = 'Very competitive' M = 3.88, SD = 1.64).

4 Results

4.1 Preliminary analyses

A correlation analysis was conducted including the dependent variables (enjoyment, interest, motivation, and social sharing), demographic variables (age, gender), and performance variables (score) to isolate potential covariates of interest (see Table 1). Only gender and score were significantly related to interest and enjoyment, respectively, and so were used as covariates in all further analyses.

4.2 Hypothesis testing

To test the effect of social sharing and feedback type on enjoyment, interest, motivation, and desire to share the game with others, we conducted a multivariate MANOVA controlling for gender and score in the game. All cell means for all conditions can be found in Table 2. Below, we discuss each dependent variable separately using the between-subjects tests for each variable.

Motivation. There was a main effect for social sharing on motivation, $F (1, 196) = 5.34$, $p < .05$, $\eta2 = .03$. There was no main effect for feedback type on motivation, $F < 1$. There was a significant interaction such that the social score condition resulted in significantly higher than the other three conditions, $F (1, 196) = 5.10$, $p < .05$, $\eta2 = .03$.

Enjoyment. Results showed a trend towards significance in the main effect for social sharing on enjoyment, $F (1, 196) = 3.15$, $p = .08$, $\eta2 = .02$. There was a main effect of feedback type on enjoyment, $F (1, 196) = 4.59$, $p < .05$, $\eta2 = .02$. There was no significant interaction effect for enjoyment, $F (1, 196) = 1.23$, $p = .30$, $\eta2 = .006$.

Interest. There was a main effect for social sharing on interest, $F (1, 196) = 4.83$, $p < .05$, $\eta2 = .02$. There was also a main effect of feedback type on interest, $F (1, 196) = 7.54$, $p < .01$, $\eta2 = .04$. Additionally, we found a significant interaction such that social score condition was significantly higher than the other three conditions, $F (1, 196) = 8.14$, $p < .01$, $\eta2 = .04$.

Competition. There were no effects for social sharing or type of feedback on perceived competitiveness within the game, nor an interaction between social sharing or feedback type on perceived competitiveness (all $F < 1$).

5   Discussion

The current study reveals the effect of shared versus private feedback on intrinsic motivation, enjoyment and performance of a brain game. In line with our expectations, we found that *socially shared, performance based* feedback increases interest and motivation to play the game. Highest scores for both measures were found in the condition in which players received a performance-based, public form of feedback. Feedback type (performance versus completion) did not affect interest or motivation independently from social sharing. These findings suggest that interest in the game and motivation to play are likely driven by related underlying motivations.

This finding is in line with the general success of SNGs, an increasingly popular game genre, with 87 per cent of American gamers playing on social networks or casual game websites [12]. Both the popularity of SNGs, and the success of the social sharing conditions in our experiment, suggests that integrating social network functionality into brain games may engage users to play for longer periods of time, thus increasing the benefits.

That said, the underlying mechanisms at work in terms of why social sharing is so popular, are not yet known. One possible explanation for our findings is that the combination of performance-related and publicly shared feedback fosters feelings of competition that motivates players. We tested for the mediating role of competition to explain changes in intrinsic motivation, however, but did not find any support for this mechanism.

Another possible mechanism is that social sharing motivates people by fulfilling psychological needs. According to Self-Determination Theory, feedback raises intrinsic motivation when it satisfies psychological needs, including needs for competence and relatedness. Indeed, recent work suggests that game features and content can function in this way [13-15] found that playing a game in a cooperative way led to greater effort and stronger commitment to in-game goals.

While we suspect that receiving feedback about an achievement and sharing it with friends and family could raise feelings of both competence and relatedness, and thus intrinsic motivation, we did not test this hypothesis directly. In the present study, sharing a simple badge on a social network site motivated participants. The badge, in this context, may have functioned as a way to socially signal a certain type of skilled behavior. Because this was a "brain game," even completion of the game irrespective of score could be an appealing signal to others, enhancing players' feelings of connection or competence. Future research should measure the components of intrinsic motivation based on Self Determination Theory in order to disentangle the underlying mechanisms of motivation in social networks games, taking into account game content as well as context.

As a single experiment conducted with social media users, we must be caution in drawing conclusions. We recruited participants who were already online using social media. According to game research, players may fall into different categories associated with different online behaviors. The study participants, as social media users, may disproportionally represent the view of what Bartle in his taxonomy of players labels "socializers" [16]. As such, we do not know whether benefits of social sharing extend to people who are not using social media sites and other player types. Yet, the ubiquity of social media and social network games suggest the widespread nature of their appeal.

In addition, our simulated brain game was not embedded within a SNG, nor did participants play for a prolonged period of time. A logical next step would be to move beyond a simulated game and a simulated social sharing manipulation to examine how and when people actually share different types of feedback on different social networks. In future work, we suggest either using existing network data like Thom et al. [17], or surveying current players to raise the ecological validity of the study.

6   Conclusion

This is the first study to experimentally test whether socially shared feedback within an existing social network affects intrinsic motivation to play and enjoyment of a brain game. The findings inform the design of successful, engaging brain games and other cognitive health based apps and games, by suggesting the advantages of situating them within existing social networks. Results suggest that there is powerful motivation to share performance based feedback within an existing social network, and that this motivation affects perceptions of the game and desire to play in the future.

References

[1]   Hardy, J., et al., *Enhancing visual attention and working memory with a web-based cognitive training program.* Mensa Research Journal, 2011. **42**(2): p. 13-20.

[2]   Nacke, L.E., A. Nacke, and C.A. Lindley, *Brain training for silver gamers: effects of age and game form on effectiveness, efficiency, self-assessment, and gameplay experience.* CyberPsychology & Behavior, 2009. **12**(5): p. 493-499.

[3]   Rabipour, S. and A. Raz, *Training the brain: Fact and fad in cognitive and behavioral remediation.* Brain and cognition, 2012. **79**(2): p. 159-179.

[4]   Deterding, S., et al. *From game design elements to gamefulness: defining gamification.* in *Proceedings of the 15th International Academic MindTrek Conference: Envisioning Future Media Environments.* 2011. ACM.

[5]   McCallum, S., *Gamification and serious games for personalized health.* Studies in health technology and informatics, 2012. **177**: p. 85-96.

[6]   Deci, E.L., R. Koestner, and R.M. Ryan, *A meta-analytic review of experiments examining the effects of extrinsic rewards on intrinsic motivation.* Psychological bulletin, 1999. **125**(6): p. 627.

[7]   Cameron, J. and W.D. Pierce, *Reinforcement, reward, and intrinsic motivation: A meta-analysis.* Review of Educational research, 1994. **64**(3): p. 363-423.

[8]   Ryan, R.M. and E.L. Deci, *Intrinsic and extrinsic motivations: Classic definitions and new directions.* Contemporary educational psychology, 2000. **25**(1): p. 54-67.

[9] Deci, E.L., R. Koestner, and R.M. Ryan, *A meta-analytic review of experiments examining the effects of extrinsic rewards on intrinsic motivation.* Psychol Bull, 1999. **125**(6): p. 627.

[10] Wang, H. and C.-T. Sun, *Game reward Systems: gaming experiences and social meanings.* Research Paper, Department of Computer Science, National Chiao Tung University, Taiwan, 2011.

[11] Vorderer, P., T. Hartmann, and C. Klimmt. *Explaining the enjoyment of playing video games: the role of competition.* in *Proceedings of the second international conference on Entertainment computing.* 2003. Carnegie Mellon University.

[12] Rozwandowicz, A. *87% of Facebook Gamers also Play on Casual Game Websites.* . Trend Report 2012 [cited 2014 April 30].

[13] Ryan, R.M., C.S. Rigby, and A. Przybylski, *The motivational pull of video games: A self-determination theory approach.* Motivation and emotion, 2006. **30**(4): p. 344-360.

[14] Tamborini, R., et al., *Defining media enjoyment as the satisfaction of intrinsic needs.* Journal of Communication, 2010. **60**(4): p. 758-777.

[15] Peng, W. and G. Hsieh, *The influence of competition, cooperation, and player relationship in a motor performance centered computer game.* Computers in Human Behavior, 2012. **28**(6): p. 2100-2106.

[16] Bartle, R., *Hearts, clubs, diamonds, spades: Players who suit MUDs.* Journal of MUD research, 1996. **1**(1): p. 19.

[17] Thom, J., D. Millen, and J. DiMicco. *Removing gamification from an enterprise SNS.* in *Proceedings of the ACM 2012 conference on Computer Supported Cooperative Work.* 2012. ACM.

Patients Should Not Be Passive! Creating and Managing Active Virtual Patients in Virtual Clinical Environments.

Wm LeRoy Heinrichs[1], Parvati Dev[2] and Dick Davies[3]

[1] Stanford University School of Medicine, Stanford, USA
(wlh@stanford.edu);
[2]Innovation in Learning, Stanford, USA
(parvati@innovationinlearning.com);
[3]Ambient Performance, London, UK
(dick.davies@ambientperformance.com)

Abstract. Games can be serious. In the case of games for medical professionals, often very serious, as they are used to train for activities that are literally lifesaving. To achieve 'suspension of disbelief' among medical professionals, a game must be realistic in terms of its' interactive elements i.e. both the objects *and* the actors in the virtual environment. The central and key actor is the patient. Given the complexity of the real world patient, then it is unsurprising that 'the patient' in most virtual environments is but a pale representation of real world patients. This paper describes work-in-progress in an already widely deployed clinical immersive environment, CliniSpace, in building believable, and as importantly manageable, real time virtual patients with an approach called 'active virtual patient management' which offers both stand-alone customisable authoring and real-time virtual patient management to deliver believable virtual patients for medical education.

Keywords: virtual patients; virtual clinical environments; virtual worlds; medical education; pathophysiological models.

1   Intro/Background

Games can be serious. In the case of games for medical professionals, often very serious, as they are used to train for activities that are literally lifesaving. To achieve suspension of belief among medical professionals in an immersive virtual environment then that experience has to be not just audio-visually immersive, it also has to be realistic in terms of its' interactive elements i.e. both the objects and the actors, in the environment. The central and key actor in both the real and the immersive medical environment is the patient. Given that the patient is a complex mix of both pathophysiology and psychology, then it is unsurprising that 'the patient' in most virtual environments is but a pale representation of actual patients and that, medical professionals quite rightly struggle to suspend belief in most virtual environments. This paper focuses on work in progress in a widely deployed clinical immersive environment – CliniSpace – that is building believable and as importantly, manageable virtual patients.

In this paper current work-in-progress in developing and building active virtual patient management tools for the CliniSpace virtual clinical environment is demonstrated and the benefits of active virtual patient management for medical education briefly explored.

2 The 'Passive' Virtual Patient in Professional Medical Education

The CliniSpace virtual clinical environment is a medical domain centric immersive 3D environment based on the renowned Unity 3D engine and deployed both as standalone and multiuser environments on a range of form factors: PC web browser and client; iPad; Android pads. In addition to realistic clinical environments i.e. wards, medical equipment, etc.. it contains virtual patients. In CliniSpace these are represented by patient avatars that are underpinned by real time and complex pathophysiology models. The patient's state is not only evident through physiological measurements e.g. heart rate, blood pressure, but also through observed appearance, such as paleness and mental state.

Most [1,2] of the few virtual patient models available for deployment in virtual environments are execute only i.e. they run from start to finish and cannot be interrupted or even most cases parameterised simply at start time. Two types of virtual patient designs can be distinguished: a 'narrative' or passive structure and a 'problem-solving' or active structure. In the narrative/passive cases, the simulation represents a single medical state, often in considerable detail, and with relevant graphics, audio and visual media displaying the patient's medical condition [1]. Fewer simulations support the evolution of the 'problem-solving'/active patient's state, both with and without medical intervention. In the problem-solving/active model, one specifies both gradual changes in physiologic variables as well as a number of discrete important "states", with the patient moving from state to state based on the virtual patient's condition and on the actions taken by the learner. For a research example see Bracegirdle [6]

From this the question arises as to why 'active' should be preferred to 'passive' virtual patients? Two reasons are advanced. Firstly, 'passive' virtual patients are experienced as pale imitations of real world patients so medical professionals find it difficult to take them seriously and, secondly they can be 'learnt' and then 'gamed' by the end user. To expand on this:

- Problems with passive models - in addition to the highlighted poor end user experience already mentioned above, most professional educators are in organisational contexts that have distinctive clinical and other associated procedures that are followed for specific clinical situations. They therefore need the clinical environment and virtual patients to be customisable in order to be able to train for local requirements. Offering virtual patient models that 'don't quite fit with our procedures' undermines credibility;

- Gaming the game – simple execute-only models can be learnt and then 'gamed' by the user over a period of time. They have a repetitive and thus predictable nature and performance. They are then viewed as not sufficiently realistic and dismissed as 'simply games'. Once played and their properties experienced, repeating 'play' again-and-again is not compelling.

In response to these issues the approach taken in CliniSpace has been to take the dynamic patient engine - DynaPatients ^{TM} - they already have and to open it up to professional end-users by offering both simple-to-use standalone authoring tools AND to enable the running virtual patient model to be adjusted by the scenario facilitator in real-time. In practice this firstly, enables the scenario controller to rapidly 'tweak' the scenario prior to run-time so changing various elements of the scenario, and secondly, by adjusting the running virtual patient model in real-time, the scenario controller is able to alter the original course of the scenario in response to real-time activities and happenings in the immersive environment. The sequence, severity and resolution of the activities and happenings can be built dynamically into the scenarios [3]. The author's initial implementation of a dynamic implementation in virtual patients – DynaPatients ^{TM} - was with the game platform, *OLIVE* [4] with the clinical management of virtual patients with Sarin poisoning and with trauma-induced hypovolemic shock as the scenario topics. The next stage of development was with the Unity-based CliniSpace platform. The next section explores in outline rapid authoring and real-time management on the current CliniSpace Unity-based platform.

3 Rapid Authoring and Real-time Management of Virtual Patients in a Virtual Clinical Environment

The opening question posed in this paper was: How can we offer believable and manageable virtual patients in a virtual environment? In terms of the user experience, firstly the virtual patient's baseline observations, e.g., vital signs must be easily identified and clustered on a typical viewing screen for rapid monitoring. Next, access to the dynamic patient's physiology must be rapid and virtual patient responses rapid, too. Both external and internal changes such as appearance to an intervention, or a change in blood pressure with fluid or drug administration are expected. And secondly, the ability to author cases of increasing complexity, with changed order of interventions, and with various outcomes is now possible with rapid authoring and real-time management by 'medical educators, not just computer scientists' [5]. In other words, both the patient and the environment must be amenable to answer the opening question.

CliniSpace offers authoring of the clinical environment and the *in silico* virtual patient via two routes to provide both pre-run time and real time management: a) Offline & Stand Alone– via the CliniSpace Authoring Tool; b) Online & in Real Time – via the Facilitator role in CliniSpace. To now examine these routes in turn:

CliniSpace provides a stand-alone set-up and authoring tool. This tool:

a)   Parameterises and sets triggers in the default virtual patient pathophysi-
     ological model in the
         CliniSpace virtual clinical environment
b)   Sets up various physical aspects of the CliniSpace environment e.g.
     rooms, equipment, dialogue, imaging graphics, etc.

and then loads them via a simple file upload into the live single or multiuser
CliniSpace environment. Each CliniSpace virtual clinical experience can therefore be
individualised for the end user(s) by the author/facilitator to link to a specific educational requirement. As an example (Fig. 1) the 'patient state interface' sets up the
parameters to the patient's initial clinical state.

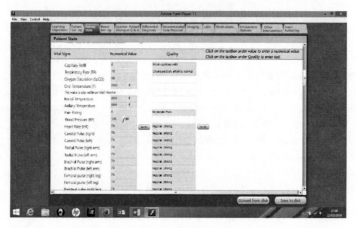

Fig. 1. Patient State Tab in CliniSpace. (Source: CliniSpace, IIL)

Further interfaces set up the patient hospital room with the objects to be visible at
the beginning of a case, medications available to be administered, imaging to be or-
dered and viewed, intravenous options, etc..

To add realism to the 'patient', an Event Authoring function offers a range of functionality that allows the author to setup and manage events in Clinispace. Multiple
conditions (Flags) can be added to a procedure to deliver a virtual patient clinical
response. For example, the administration of a *combination* of drugs to lower a patient's heart rate. Event Authoring is a key and new component of the CliniSpace
stand-alone set-up application and consists of the following elements: Procedures –
general, medications and intravenous options Attributes – vital signs, animations,
sounds, texts, states. Flags – conditions that are added to Procedures Transitions –
Start and Stop conditions

The other key aspect of virtual patient management is real-time facilitator intervention. (Fig. 2)

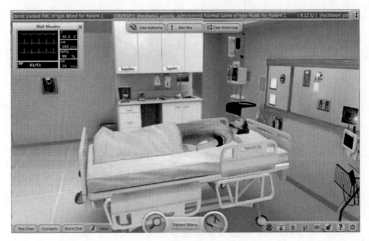

Fig. 2. Facilitator View – note Facilitator Menu at Top on Screen. (Source: CliniSpace, IIL)

In this the running patient model can be moved forward in time, stopped and re-started, etc... This real-time function is particularly useful, for example, after administering a drug such as an antibiotic which, in the real world, would naturally take some time to have effect. In this case the scenario can be moved on a number of hours in real time by the facilitator, so enabling a case scenario to be completed.

Taken together this dual active management functionality within CliniSpace – offline stand-alone authoring and real-time facilitator intervention – provides active virtual patient management.

4   The Benefits of Active Virtual Patient Management

In summary, the benefits of active virtual patient management in CliniSpace are threefold and closely linked to the perspectives of the users. The users are firstly, the medical professional undergoing training, secondly, the medical educator and thirdly, and more generally, the community in which medical professionals practice. For the medical professional undergoing training the custom stand-alone and real-time adjusted models make the scenario more realistic and so professionally more realistic and so acceptable. For the medical educator the simulation therefore has a better chance of achieving its objective of being an immersive environment that is a small 'step' from the real environments that the student will encounter in the real world enabling the transfer of their expertise more readily. For the community, more medical professionals trained in realistic clinical settings are by definition necessary for good patient care.

5   References:

[1] Dev, P., Heinrichs, W L., Youngblood, P., Kung, S., Cheng, R., Kusumoto, L. MS, Hendrick, A.: Virtual Patient Model for Multi-Person Virtual Medical Environments. AMIA Annual Symp Proc. 2007: pg.181–185 http://www. ncbi.nlm.nih.gov/pmc/articles/PMC2655782/ abstract.(2008)

[2] Bearman, M., Cesnik, B, Liddell, M.: Random comparison of 'virtual patient' models in the context of teaching clinical communication skills. Medical Education Volume 35, Issue 9, pg. 824–832, (2013)

[3]

[4] Heinrichs, W L., Kung, S-Y., Dev, P.: Design and Implementation of Rule-based Medical Models: An *In*

[5] *Silico* Patho-physiological Trauma Model for Hypovolemic Shock/ Proceedings, MMVR2008, Long Beach, CA Jan. 2008; IOS Press pg. 159-164.(2008)

[6] Heinrichs, W L., Harter, P., Youngblood P., Kusumoto, L., Dev, P.: Training Healthcare Personnel for Mass Casualty Incidents in a Virtual Emergency Department; VED II. 2010 Pre-hospital and Disaster Medicine, 25(5):422–434 (2010)

[7] Talbot, T.B., Sagae, K., John, B., Rizzo, A.A.: Sorting Out the Virtual Patient: How to Exploit Artificial Intelligence, Game Technology and Sound Educational Practices to Create Engaging Role-Playing Simulations, International Journal of Gaming and Computer-Mediated Simulations (IJGCMS), 4(3), 1-19 (2012)

[8] Bracegirdle, L., Chapman, S.: Programmable Patients: Simulation of Consultation Skills in a Virtual Environment. Bio-Algorithms and Med-Systems. Vol.6, No.11. pp 111-115. [2010]

The Opinions of People in the Netherlands over 65 on Active Video Games: a Survey Study

Annerieke Heuvelink[1], Erwin C. P. M. Tak[1], Nico L. U. van Meeteren[1,2,3]

[1]TNO Healthy Living, The Netherlands, [2]Center for Care Technology Research, Maastricht, the Netherlands, [3]CAPHRI, Maastricht University, the Netherlands
{Annerieke.Heuvelink, Erwin.Tak, Nico.vanMeeteren}@tno.nl

Abstract. Active video games can potentially support healthy aging by stimulating physical activity. We conducted a survey study amongst 482 Dutch people over 65 to learn their opinions and found that many are not interested in playing active video games. Participants that have played them like and interact more with ordinary (computer) games and computers than those who have not. We hypothesize that in order for active video games to be used for health enhancement more promotional efforts are required to let more people experience active video gaming and to increase awareness on its use as physical activity.

1   Introduction

In recent years health enhancing games for seniors have increasingly gained attention. Research has shown that active video games (AVG) – games that are played by moving body parts - can contribute to good health of seniors. The physical activity required to play AVG can improve physical function (such as balance) and initial results indicate a positive effect on cognition [1, 2] and on a social-emotional level [3].

For AVG to reach its potential in contributing to healthy aging it is required that seniors (are willing to) play AVG. At the moment little is known about the opinion of seniors about AVG. Most information stems from small pilot studies that suffer from participation bias. An exception in the Netherlands is a survey by broadcasting station Max in 2012 amongst its members about 'Interactive and Serious Games'. 986 People over 65 participated and answered questions like: "How attractive are AVG?" and "Would you prefer AVG or sports?" The results are descriptive of the general attitude of Dutch seniors. However, because few participant details were collected, the study failed to provide any rational behind people's opinions. Therefore our objective was to conduct a survey study amongst people over 65 to investigate their opinions about AVG and determinants of that opinion. In particular, we asked whether they knew and used AVG, reasons for them to (start to) play or not (start to) play AVG, and how they would like to play AVG. To interpret the results we enquired after individual characteristics (e.g. gender, education level, overall health) and their attitude and behavior towards physical activity, playing (computer) games and using the computer.

2 Method

People over 65 were approached in 2013 via an (existing) online research panel recruited from the general Dutch population. Of the 3106 people approached, 482 people (16%) completed and returned the survey within a week. All data was – after check of completeness, correctness and distributions – converted in information via conservative regular descriptive statistics (like counts, percentages, means, SDs). Next we compared the participants that stated to have played AVG with those that did not using chi-square and t-tests (2-tailed) to identify potential determinants of AVG play.

3 Results

3.1 Participants

Of the participants 64% were male and 96% were of Dutch origin. The mean age was 72 years (SD 4, range 66-88 years), 84% had children and 74% grandchildren. Participants were equally low (39%), secondary (30%) and highly educated (31%). 70% lived with a partner or family, 11% lived in a senior complex. Subjective health was for 55% good / very good; for 34% not good/bad; and for 11% poor / very poor. 11% of participants used a walking aid, of which 85% outdoors only.

3.2 Acquaintance and Experiences

Of the participants 29% stated they have never heard of AVG. Of the group who stated to have heard of AVG 18% (n=60) reported to have played AVG: we will refer to them as the AVG-players. 15% Reported to have access to an AVG system, through their own household (8%) or through others (7%). Access seemed not necessary nor associated with having played AVG: 56% of the AVG-players reported to have no access. Of those that stated to have access through their household 61% were AVG-players vs 30% of the people who stated to know a person with an AVG system.

Of the AVG-players the majority (72%) stated they (really) liked it, only 9% did not like it (at all). Of the group that stated to have never heard of AVG 98% reported that they were not planning to play AVG anytime the coming six months; of the group that had heard about AVG 12% did state to plan to play AVG the coming six months. Of the 43 people who reported to have played AVG and to (really) like it 22 people (51%) stated to plan to play AVG the coming six months.

3.3 Motivations and Barriers

Table 1 provides an overview of the reasons selected by the participants as the main motivation to (start to) play AVG.

Table 1. Main reason participants selected to (start to) play AVG (single-choice):

To be physically active	28%	To challenge myself	4%
Other reason (particularly 'I do not want to play')	23%	Useful pastime	2%
To have fun	16%	To meet others	1%
To try something new	13%	To get out of the house	1%
To be mentally active	7%	Competition with others	0,5%
Fun pastime	5%		

We found some differences between AVG-players and non-players. The AVG-players mentioned as main motivations 'To be physically active' (40% vs 26%) and 'To have fun' (28% vs 14%), while 'To try something new' was hardly mentioned by those that had played AVG (3% vs 15%).

Table 2 provides an overview of the reasons selected by all the participants as the main motivation to not (start to) play AVG.

Table 2. Main reason participants selected to not (start to) play AVG (single-choice):

Not interested	26%	Don't think it will be fun	2%
No added value	12%	Don't have the space for it	2%
Don't want to spend money on a system	11%	Don't want to learn something new	2%
Already physically active enough	9,5%	Don't know where to do it	1%
Too busy	9%	Don't think they'll be good at it	1%
Don't want to go somewhere	5%	System too difficult	1%
Don't like games	5%	Forgetful	0,5%
Don't think are able physically	4%	Don't know anybody to do it with	0,5%
Other reason	4%	Don't like the people that do it	0%
Afraid to fall	3%	Can't see well enough	0%
Don't know how to do it	2,5%		

Again we found differences between AVG-players and non-players. The AVG-players reported two main reasons for not wanting to play, namely that they do not want to spend the money on a system at home (18% vs 10%) and that they do not want to go anywhere to do it (15% vs 3%).

To the question 'From who would you take advice regarding playing AVG' 48% of the non-players answered 'Nobody' vs 20% from the AVG-players. If the non-players reported to be willing to take advice than mostly from (grand)children (26% vs 50%) and from a doctor / physical therapist (25% vs 35%).

3.4 Game Play Preferences

To the question: 'Where do you want to play AVG?' the vast majority (91%) answered at home; 12% stated they want to play outside their home.

Table 3. Reasons people selected to play at home or outside their home (multiple-choice):

Reason to play at home	%	Reason to play outside the home	%
Having exclusive access at any time	39	Easier to play with others	49
Playing in their own environment	35	Needing help with the system	30
Not wanting to travel to the activity	30	No opportunity for system @ home	28
Only wanting to play by myself or with household member	20	Getting out of the house	21
		Other reason	12
Other reason (not wanting to play)	15	Risk of falling at home	7

To the question: 'How would you like to play AVG?' 76% selected 'By myself' and 28% 'With others'. These numbers are significantly different for the AVG-players: of them more than half (57%) selected 'By myself' and 'With others' (55%).

Table 4. Reasons people selected to play alone or with others (multiple-choice)

Reason to play alone	%	Reason to play with others	%
Possibility to play at any suitable time	52	Enjoying time spend with others	53
Playing in their own way and pace	44	Enjoying competition	31
Other reason (not wanting to play)	16	Not self-motivated enough	29
Only interested in self improvement	12	Help available in case of falls	12
Not knowing anybody to play with	11	Needing help with the system	10
Not wanting to look like a fool	7	Other reason	7

3.5 Determinants

Self-reported players of AVG did not significantly differ from non-players on the individual characteristics of gender, education level and subjective health. Also no significant differences were found for physical activity: both groups stated to be equally physically active throughout their lives and to currently exercise a similar amount according to the Dutch healthy exercise norm, Fitnorm and Combinorm [4].

We did find significant differences in the reported attitudes and behavior of partic-ipants towards playing (computer) games and using the computer. Of all participants 33% stated to not like it (at all) to play ordinary, non-computer games; 48% stated to like it (a lot). Those numbers differ significantly ($P<0.001$) for the AVG-players: of them only 10% stated to not like it (at all) and more than 70% stated to like it (a lot). AVG-players also reported more frequently that they had played non-computer games in the last six months (77% vs 61%). Moreover, AVG-players stated to like to work with computers significantly more than the non-players (4.4 vs. 3.9 on a scale of 1 = not at all to 5 = a lot, $p<0.001$). They also stated to use the computer more (18 vs. 15 hours per week, $p<0.05$) and to play more computer games (6 vs. 4 hours per week, $p<0.05$). The type of computer games the participants stated to play the most were single-player casual games such as Minesweeper, FreeCell, Solitaire, and Angry Birds.

4 Discussion and Conclusion

Although 'To be physically active' is mentioned as main AVG-play motivation by the participants, our study shows that the AVG-players amongst the participants are typified by an increased preference of computers and (computer) games. It thus seems plausible that the current senior views AVG mainly as a computer game and not as a way to be physically active. However, care should be taken in generalizing the findings from this study to the general public. First because of the relative small number of participants that actually stated to have played AVG. Second because the participants might not be representative of the general Dutch population, despite the fact van the online panel was recruited from it. In particular, 58% of the 3104 people approached was male and of the participants 64% was male. In contrast only 48% of the Dutch population of 72 years old (the average age of the participants) was male in 2013 [5].

In order for AVG to reach its potential in aiding with the challenges of an aging population the opinions of Dutch people over 65 about AVG need to change. Foremost more seniors have to learn about the existence of AVG and their potential health benefits. Given the difference in opinions about AVG between AVG-players vs non-players, we propose in particular to increase positive play experiences among seniors.

Acknowledgement

We thank Anja Langefeld for her help with the statistical analysis. This study was funded by TNO, the Dutch ministry of Economic Affairs, Agriculture and Innovation, VitaValley and the Noaber Foundation (ELI-Co 051.01284).

References

[1] Hall, A.K., Chavarria, E., Maneeratana, V., Chaney, B.H., Bernhardt, J.M.: Health Benefits of Digital Videogames for Older Adults: A Systematic Review of the Literature. Games for Health Journal 1(6), 402-410 (2012)

[2] Larsen, L.H., Schou, L., Lund, H.H., Langberg, H.: The Physical Effect of Exergames in Healthy Elderly—A Systematic Review. Games for Health Journal 2(4), 205-212 (2013)

[3] Wollersheim D, Merkes M, Shields N, Liamputtong, P., Walis, L., Reynolds, F. Koh, L.C.: Physical and psychosocial effects of Wii video game use among older women. International Journal of Emerging Technologies and Society 8(2), 85-98 (2010)

[4] Kemper, H.G.C, Ooijendijk, W.T.M, Stiggelbout, M.: Consensus over de Nederlandse Norm voor Gezond Bewegen. Tijdschrift Sociale Gezondheidszorg 78, 180-183 (2000)

[5] http://statline.cbs.nl

Tactical Forms:
Classification of Applied Games for Game Design

Micah Hrehovcsik[1], Joeri Taelman[2], Joep Janssen[3] and Niels Keetels[1]

[1]HKU University of the Arts Utrecht, Hilversum, the Netherlands
micah.hrehovcsik@hku.nl
niels.keetels@hku.nl
[2]Utrecht University, Utrecht, the Netherlands
j.g.g.taelman@students.uu.nl
[3]De Hoogstraat Revalidatie
j.janssen@dehoogstraat.nl

Abstract. Entertainment game genres provide game designers with a taxonomy of known sets of mechanics, which are used as a foundation to design games. Serious games taxonomy in comparison do not provide the same kind of design knowledge. For this reason, we adopted a way of classifying serious games into four categories by tactical form, or the way the game is deployed in a certain context to achieve its primary purpose. Central to this paper is the discussion of our extended tactical from termed adaptive. DJ Fiero, a game designed to reha-bilitate children with ABI (Acquired Brain Injury), is used as a case study to examine how the adaptive form fits the current sociopolitical and economic design challenges of the Dutch healthcare domain.

Keywords: serious games · game design · theory · taxonomy · genre · healthcare · rehabilitation

1 Introduction

The development and design of games applied to fields such as healthcare, govern-ment, defense, education, research. etc., are increasingly multidisciplinary. These *applied games*[1] benefit from the combined expertise of game designers, subject matter experts, researchers, and input from the target audience [1] [2]. Game designers in particular are challenged with the task of designing the balancing between a game's purpose, sustainability and game-play experience [3]. They become "applied" game designers, who are expected to connect game design activity, game design principles, methods and processes to a meaningful application in real-life [4]. Applied game designers, trained and educated originally as entertainment game designers, must rely on operational knowledge from the entertainment industry [5], an important aspect of which concerns itself with game genres and their taxonomy.

---

[1] The term 'applied game' indicates games designed with a purpose other than entertainment.

In general, the purpose of game taxonomy varies according to a parties interests or worldviews. The current video game genres originated from game journalism and the games industry to provide product information about the games [6]. Players have come to expect certain sets of conventions from these genres [7]. Game genres and taxonomy is also used by game researchers, who study the historical development of a game genre or explore the role of games from a sociological approach or as cultural phenomenon [6]. Serious game advocates use taxonomy as a way to "get all parties on the same page" and "provide a snapshot of the current state of serious games industry" [8]. Game designers use genres to identify a "system", where a set of mechanics have become so well-known that games use most or all the set [9]. If a game designer wishes to make a rigorous analysis of a game's mechanics he or she can use *game design patterns* to communicate more specific aspects of a game's design [10]. This allows a designer to base the design of an entertainment game on a genre or a game mechanic.

However, entertainment genres are not as relevant to applied game design. And some game mechanics (e.g. randomness, time compression, perfect communication, etc.) commonly used for entertainment are even considered undesirable [7]. Since the primary goal of any *applied game* is the use and usefulness of its game activity outside the domain of the game itself [4]. An applied game could be any genre or have any game mechanic as long as the game achieves its desired goal(s) [7], i.e. therapy, persuasion, training, education, data exchange, human computing, etc. While there are several applied game taxonomies, which ones are relevant to the operational knowledge of applied game design?

The aim of this paper is to introduce a classification of applied games by *tactical form* or the way the game is deployed in a certain context to achieve its primary purpose. We distinguish between four kinds of *tactical forms*: *transmissive, aggregative, collaborative*, and *adaptive*. While this way of classification is not new, we do propose the additional *adaptive* category. To elaborate on this new category we use the applied game DJ Fiero as a case study. DJ Fiero is being developed for patients with ABI (Acquired Brain Injury) by De Hoogstraat[2] and the HKU University of the Arts Utrecht[3]. Besides its primary purpose, DJ Fiero also faces difficult design challenges that are a result of the current sociopolitical and economic recession in the Netherlands. Designing DJ Fiero as an *adaptive* applied game is a part of our efforts to overcome these challenges.

2 Game Taxonomy

Categorization by genre has proven a useful way of looking at literature and film [11]. And when faced with a domain like games it is only natural to devise a structured approach to their study. Most likely the first categorization of games in general was devised by Callois [12], who organized games by agon (competition), alea (chance),

---

[2] http://www.dehoogstraat.nl/
[3] http://gi.hku.nl/

mimicry (role-playing), and Ilinx (sensation that alters perception). These categories have been extended to include fellowship (cooperation), narrative (unfolding a story), expression (sand-box play), submission (mindless pastime), challenge (obstacle courses) and discovery (exploration and charting new territory) [13].

The non-systematic approach to genres taken by journalism and adopted by the games industry allows developers and publishers to share a common language [14]. Players too, have certain expectations from a genre, and may be disappointed if these expectations are not met [9] [15]. The games industry benefits from this predictability and consistency genres offers, because it removes the inherent risk that occurs when exploring new combinations of game mechanics [15]. However, the approaches used to structure taxonomy of digital games has faced several challenges. One of these being digital games approached and studied as a medium for story-telling [6]. Another is that these games are not a single medium, but many media [16]. Finally, games in a genre evolve making old sets of game mechanics obsolete [17]. These issues have made traditional approaches to the study of digital games useless [17] [16].

Crawford [18] proposed one of the first genre based taxonomy of digital games to "illuminate common factors that link families of games" and identify unexplored areas of game design [18]. Wolf [11] proposes a classification based primarily on interactivity, which can be combined with iconography and thematic genres (like those from films). His classification of game interactivity include categories, i.e. abstract, adaption, adventure, card games, capturing, collecting, artificial life, etc. Other approaches, provide tools to describe how different categories of games enable different experiences of play and their connection with historical, social and technological 'situations' [19]. Similarly, Lindley's [20] taxonomy is a tool for that allows for specific classification using four dimensions, which determine a game's affinity based on: 1) it being Ludic, Narrative, or Simulation; 2) its randomness or chance; 3) its fictional content 4) and its virtual and physical contrast. Björk, Lundgren and Holopainen [6] proposed the use of game mechanics to identify the common components constituting a genre. Their approach aimed to translate game mechanics into *game design patterns* which could be used for analysis (e.g. structural analysis or playtesting) or for game design (e.g. idea generation, problem-solving, communication, developing concepts). They support the game design patterns with a framework to describe all kinds of games from various perspectives (e.g. holistic, temporal, boundary, structural) [10].

Current applied game taxonomies are either categorized by domain or market (i.e. military, government, healthcare, etc.) or purpose (i.e. Advergames, Exergaming, Health and Medicine Games, etc.) [21]. Some of these taxonomies are extended to include technology platform, target audience, and learning principles [22]. An approach taken by Alverez and Djaouti [21] combines the strengths of previous classification systems by classifying games according to their "serious-related" and "game-related" characteristics. Their G/P/S model provides a tool for subject matter experts (e.g. teachers) to identify and classify applied games.

3   Applied Game Design and Genre

An applied game designer, like a game designer, is an advocate for the player and the player experience [14] [23]. He or she works with formal game elements (e.g. systems, rules, internal relationships, objects, boundaries and outcome), and through a series of design decisions eventually creates a game system that determines the player's available choices, actions and ultimately the player experience [14]. An applied game designer connects the formal game elements, the player's choices, actions and game experience to the real-life goal(s) of an applied game. His or her biggest challenge is balancing the applied game's purpose, sustainability and gameplay experience. Ideally, a game designer is not limited by technology or genre, and capable of designing all kinds of games [24], while an applied game designer is not limited to a specific domain of expertise.

Genre knowledge allows a game designer a means to identify well-known and successful sets of game mechanics. Many games find their original concept rooted in a genre's predefined game mechanics [9] [7], because their game mechanics are inherently fun [15]. However, game designers criticize the use of genre, because it restricts creativity by being too reliant on tried and true design solutions [14] [15] or promoting "this is the way this genre does it" kind of dominant thinking [9].

Applied game genres primarily explore the domains or purpose of a game, but do not identify well known and successful sets of applied game mechanics for a designer to draw from. Furthermore, applied game designers cannot depend on entertainment genres to support their design, where some common game mechanics used in entertainment purposes would have undesirable results in an applied game [7]. The lack of tried and true design solutions means designers must explore new combinations of game mechanics, which makes making applied games risky to develop [15]. While tools like *game design patterns* [10] do not offer patterns related to the contextual situation (e.g. hospital, school, company, etc.) [3] [7] that applied game designers must consider it their game's design.

4   Tactical Forms

4.1   Theory

The theory presented here was originally developed as lecture material for HKU University of the Arts Utrecht game design students. The purpose of the material was to offer students with a way to differentiate applied games and identify the challenges of designing an applied game [25]. One of these challenges is the design of an applied game's sustainability [3] [25].

Tactical form is our term to describe the way an applied game's deployment is designed for a certain context. The term is derived from van Roessel's and van Mastrigt's [4] argument for the use of the term *applied game*. *"Application,"* they argue. "Refers to the tactical use and usefulness of the game activity outside the domain of the game itself. In other words, application does not so much refer to the game itself, but rather to the way the game is deployed in certain contexts." In our definition, *tactical* refers the design considerations about the game's deployment in a certain context. While the *form* refers to design patterns used by the game for deployment in a certain context.

The purpose of *tactical form* is to provide a map or model that defines fundamental relationships that exist in the design of an applied game's deployment. In any given applied game deployment there are four elements. The first elements in concerned with the stakeholders or the party responsible for determining the goal(s) the game. The second element is the target audience or the players for which the game has been designed. The third element is the applied game itself designed, developed and deployed to achieve predetermined a goal(s). The fourth element is a directional flow, which indicates the primary purpose of the game. The flow establishes the relationship between stakeholder, target audience, and the applied game artefact.

4.2 Taxonomy

The proposed categories of *tactical form* share similarities to categories also observed in other theories. In particular, the term and categorization of "purpose" by Duke [26] and Djaouti, Alvarez, and Jessel [27], whose use of the term *purpose* differs from taxonomies that use the same term to refer to the goal (e.g. practicing skills, cognitive problem-solving, recruitment, exergaming, etc.) of an applied game. Duke's [26] concept of *purpose* is a step in the design process towards deciding an applied game's objectives. He defines four categories of *purpose*, three of which we recognize as tactical "use" of an applied game: 1) Dialogue, the game stimulates communication about complex topics; 2) Project, the game aims to inform, educate or train; 3) Extract, the game takes opinions or information from players. 4) Motivate, the game motivates players, but is always coupled with the previously mentioned purposes.

In our theory creating motivation is an essential reason for the use of all applied games. Furthermore, unlike the other three categories it cannot be defined with the elements of a *tactical form*. Currently, we have four categories of *tactical form*, which we refer to as: *transmissive, aggregative, collaborative,* and *adaptive*. These terms were selected for being descriptive and distinguishable from similar concepts previously mentioned.

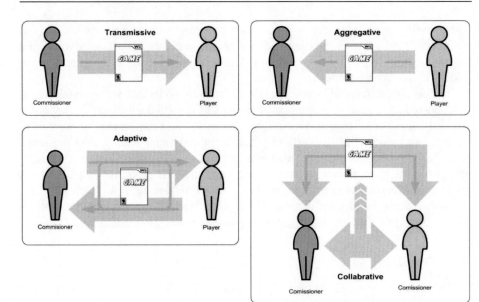

Fig. 1. The four types of *tactical forms*

Transmissive. The *transmissive tactical form* describes an applied game meant to achieve its goals by projecting or transmitting by engaging players. A commissioner's goals may aim to: educate, inform, persuade, train skills, coach, medicate, change player behavior, etc. Examples of games that follow this kind *tactical form* include: America's Army[4], Re-Mission[5], Triage Trainer[6], Darfur is Dying[7], etc. These games are usually designed as a stand-alone solution, but in some cases require supervision from a trainer, coach, teacher or therapist. These professionals act as a supervisor facilitating game sessions by controlling the context (who, where, when) the game is played, determine didactic goals, evaluating the player's progress, or relating game learning to the real-world knowledge. Players may play the game alone, a part of a community or with the help (outside of the game) of a supervisor.

Aggregative. The *aggregative tactical form* describes an applied game meant to extract or collect from player engagement to achieve its goals. A commissioner's goals may aim to: collect data, solve problems with human-computing, classify data, collect user generated content, etc. Examples of games that follow this kind *tactical form* include: Foldit[8], Phylo[9], ESP game, Google Image Labeler, etc. Players may play alone, together or through an online community.

4 http://www.americasarmy.com/
5 http://www.re-mission.net/
6 http://www.trusim.com/
7 http://www.darfurisdying.com/
8 http://fold.it/
9 http://phylo.cs.mcgill.ca/

Collaborative. The *collaborative tactical form* describes an applied game meant to create a dialogue or collaboration with participants acting as commissioners, designers and/or players. A commissioner's goals may aim to: explore and examine business challenges, inspire new perspectives, improve collaboration, co-design complex systems or future-oriented systems, policy making, etc.. Examples of games that follow this kind *tactical form* include: De Climategame[10], Deltaviewer[11], Urban Strategy[12], etc. Compared to other kinds of applied games the game artifact may be rudimentary. The game artifact may not even be "playable" on its own and need supervision from a game master, game designer or consultant. These professionals act as a supervisor facilitating game sessions by acting as mediators and event hosts. The player-participants may decide their own goals or even come together to design their own game to play.

Adaptive. The *adaptive tactical form* describes an applied game meant to extract from player engagement and project through player engagement to achieve its goals. A commissioner's goals may aim to: adapt the game to the individual player, regulate difficulty levels, change the relationship between professional and player (e.g. therapist and patient vs. game master and player), allow real-time interventions based on real-time interactions, tailor workloads to increase effectiveness and efficiency, etc. The player and the professional-user take advantage of the interaction through the game it to the individual. There is a lack of examples of games that follow this kind of *tactical form* and for that reason we use DJ Fiero as a case study in the following section. The *adaptive tactical form* is our contribution to previously discussed theories on the applied game deployment.

5   DJ Fiero

5.1   Context

As the Dutch government makes cuts to funding healthcare, doctors and therapists must find efficient ways to treat their patients and maintain quality healthcare [28]. Both the HKU University of the Arts Utrecht and De Hoogstraat consider applied games as a way to make healthcare more efficient and effective. Therapists' confrontation with game technology and design holds potential for inspiring new ideas for therapeutic training [29]. De Hoogstraat has been a forerunner in The Netherlands in using COTS (Commercial off-the-shelf) videogames and gaming hardware as part of their children's rehabilitation programs for training relevant motor, socio-emotional and cognitive skills. However, the drawback of using COTS games remains that they have not been designed with therapeutic outcomes in mind, so therapists at De Hoogstraat often worked with hardware modifications or improvised meta-games for

---

[10] http://climategame.nl/
[11] http://www.deltaviewer.nl/
[12] https://www.tno.nl

interventions to have the desired effect. Moreover, the therapeutic needs of children with ABI vary to such an extent that much greater demands are required from a game in terms of flexibility and customization, making COTS less than optimal solutions.

For these reasons, researchers at De Hoogstraat have joined HKU University of the Arts Utrecht to create a new applied game that not only addresses these issues but also affords previously unattainable efficiencies. The aim is to combine knowledge about therapy, healthcare, and research with game design and development to create a game with the intrinsic requirements of both healthcare and gaming for making purposeful interventions. DJ Fiero is the result of this collaboration and conceived under the assumption that the entertainment value of the game will offer the patient: 1) the motivation to train for a longer periods of time and more frequently, shifting their focus to in-game dynamics and performance rather than highly repetitive fitness-like exercises. 2) a better understanding of the trainable disabilities; 3) and a consistent stream of data showing improvements over time.

Game

The theme of DJ Fiero is based on a modern disco-club, putting the player in the role of a DJ in front of an abstract crowd. The task of the DJ is to give a concert. The game uses the theme because it fits closely to the mechanics of the game's dance-like movements. And based on research conducted with the target audience, the theme also agreed with the patients' perception of a DJ.

The goal of the game, is for the player (patient) to complete a concert (consisting of a number exercises) and increase the size and excitement of their in-game audience for a high-score. The player accomplishes this by matching his or her extremities to in-game target positions facilitated by the Microsoft Kinect. A 3D silhouette of a human figure with six points symbolizing the extremities (the head, the torso, two hands and two feet) represent the player in-game (see Fig.2). The player uses the six points to determine what the Kinect detects. In this way the player meets the challenge to move their body into different positions to match their reference points with targets as they appear.

The player starts a game session with a game environment that offers little interaction. When players move their body into positions to match game targets, players earn points. Used as a game mechanism to encourage progression, these points can then be used as currency to increase the excitement or growth of the audience during a concert. As a player progresses the game environment becomes increasingly more interactive and rewarding.

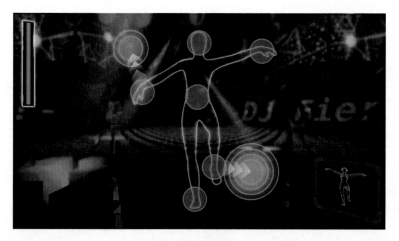

Fig. 2: DJ Fiero

Function

Patients challenged by the core game-play move their impaired and unimpaired extremities. A rehabilitation therapist can configure DJ Fiero from a back-end application changing the game-play to emphasize movement of the impaired extremities.

To conceal repetition of these exercises additional challenging game-play is blended into the game session. A typical game session exists of predetermined amount of time and exercises. The therapist can also adjust exercises to fit the rehabilitation process and accommodate individual patients by controlling settings for the range of motion (e.g. small, middle and full). Data concerning the patient's therapeutic progression is also collected, and available to therapists in the back-end. Using this data therapists can then remotely adjust the therapy (e.g. increase difficulty) allowing patients to continue their therapy outside the rehabilitation clinic.

DJ Fiero's Tactical Form

The current applied game taxonomy would classify the game DJ Fiero in the *domain* of healthcare and as a game for health. The *purpose* would have it categorized as rehabitainment or cybertherpy [8]. The *target audience* would be children with ABI (Acquired Brain Injury) using a PC (with online connectivity) and a Kinect as its *technology*. The *game-play* of DJ Fiero could be roughly categorized under the entertainment genre of a music game and/or exergame.

DJ Fiero's *tactical form* classification is *adaptive*, because it has the ability to project and extract goals through the game. The *adaptive* aspect of the game begins by the therapist determining the content (e.g. relevant therapeutic exercises) projected to the patient. The player receives this content translated through the game into game-play. Players provide real-time data about their progress and movements during the game. Therapists can use this extracted information in various ways, i.e. adjust the therapy on-the-fly to keep the game from being too easy or too hard or remotely monitor and coach the players at home. Finally, the therapist can use player data to help inform the patient about his or her disability, which can then be used by the patient to improve their ability to play the game. An analysis with *tactical form* would also include the ulterior purposes of the applied game's stakeholders. For example, DJ Fiero's *tactical form* could significantly lower the cost of one-on-one contact with the therapist, prevent patients at home from becoming isolated, and even stimulate the social-emotional environment with family and peers.

6   Conclusion

Until genres and their patterns connect with specific verifiable real-world effects for applied game design, efforts should be made to support applied game designers with the complexities of designing applied games. Looking at applied games by their *tactical form* offers an interesting perspective to game designers. Where the focus is on how a game is designed and developed for application to a certain context. Using the aforementioned *tactical forms* (*transmissive, aggregative, collaborative*, and *adaptive*) provides game designers paradigms to be used as foundations for designing the deployment aspect of a game.

DJ Fierro, though still in development, promises to provide an interesting example of the *adaptive tactical form*, which has the potential of allowing therapists to ensure quality care but also support therapists in becoming more efficient. Currently, multiple DJ Fiero prototypes have been play-tested by ABI patients at the rehabilitation center De Hoogstraat, who have responded well to the game. Once a version of DJ Fiero with all core features has been developed, it will allow therapists to gather data about therapy with games in a way never done before and potentially become a valuable research tool as well as a therapeutic one.

7   References

[1] N. Keetels, Designing Games for Children's Rehabilitation, Bournemouth University, 2012.

[2] P. M. Kato, "The Role of the Researcher in Making Serious Games for Health," in *Serious Games for Healthcare: Applications and Implications*, S. Arnab, I. Dunwell and K. Debattista, Eds., Hershey, PA, IGI Global, 2012, pp. 213-231.

[3] M. Hrehovcsik and L. v. Roessel, "Using Vitruvius as a Framework for Applied Game Design," in *Games for Health: Proceedings of the 3rd european conference on gaming and playful interaction in health care*, Springer, 2013, pp. 131-152.

[4] L. v. Roessel and J. v. Mastrigt, "Collaboration and Team Composition in Applied Game Creation Processes," 2011.

[5] C. Totten, "Teaching Serious Game App Design Through Client-based Projects," DiGRA 2013: DeFragging Game Studies, 2013.

[6] S. Björk, S. Lundgren and J. Holopainen, "Game Design Patterns," in *Level Up Conference Proceedings*, Utrecht, 2003.

[7] D. Michael and S. Chen, Serious Games: Games that Educate, Train, and Inform, Course Technology , Cengage Learning, 2006.

[8] B. Sawyer and P. Smith, "Serious Games Taxonomy," 2008. [Online]. Available: http://www.dmill.com/presentations/serious-games-taxonomy-2008.pdf.

[9] L. Pulsipher, Game Design: How to Create Video and Tabletop Games, Start to Finish, McFarland, 2012.

[10] S. Bjork and J. Holopainen, Patterns in Game Design, Charles River Media, 2004.

[11] M. J. P. Wolf, "Genre and the Video Game," in *The Medium of the Video Game*, M. J. P. Wolf, Ed., University of Texas Press, 2001, pp. 113-134.

[12] R. Caillois, Man, Play and Games, University of Illinois Press, 1961.

[13] M. LeBlanc, "Formal Design Tools: Emergent Complexity, Emergent Narrative.," 2000. [Online]. Available: http://algorithmancy.8kindsoffun.com/gdc2000.ppt.

[14] T. Fullerton, C. Swain and S. Hoffman, Game Design Workshop: Designing, Prototyping, and Playtesting Games, CMP Books , 2004.

[15] N. McKenzie, "Nuturing Lateral Leaps in Game Design," in *Games, Learning and Soceity: Learning and Meaning in the Digital Age*, C. Steinkuehler, K. Squire and S. Barab, Eds., Cambridge University Press, 2012, pp. 49-74.

[16] E. Aarseth, "Computer Game Studies, Year One," *The International Journal of Computer Game Research,* 2001.

[17] D. Arsenault, "Video Game Genre, Evolution and Innovation," *Eludamos Journal for Computer Game Culture,* pp. 149-176, 2009.

[18] C. Crawford, Chris Crawford on Game Design, 1st ed., New Riders, 2003.

[19] R. Klevjer, "Genre blindness," 2006. [Online]. Available: http://www.digra.org/hc11-rune-klevjer-genre-blindness/.

[20] C. A. Lindley, "Gamasutra - Features - Game Taxonomies: A High Level Framework for Game Analysis and Design," 2003. [Online]. Available: http://www.gamasutra.com/view/feature/2796/game_taxonomies_a_high_level_.php.

[21] J. Alverez and D. Djaouti, "Une taxinomie des Serious Games dédiés au secteur de la santé," in *L'application des jeux vidéo à la médecine et à la surveillance*, 2008.

[22] R. Ratan and U. Ritterfeld, "Classifying Serious Games," in *Serious Games: Mechanisms and Effects*, Routledge, 2009, pp. 10-24.

[23] J. Schell, The Art of Game Design: A Book of Lenses, Morgan Kaufmann, 2008.

[24] E. Adams and A. Rollings, Fundamentals of game design, Upper Saddle River: Prentice Hall, 2007.

[25] M. Hrehovcsik, "Applied Game Design: Content, Context and Transfer," in *Proceedings of the Serious Games Conference 2014: Bridging Communities, Harnessing Technologies and Enriching Lives*, Serious Games Conference 2014, Ilsan KINTEX, Korea, Seoul, 2014.

[26] R. Duke, Gaming: The Future's Language, SAGE Publications, 1974.

[27] D. Djaouti, J. Alvarez and J.-P. Jessel, "Classifying Serious Games: the G/P/S model," in *Handbook of Research on Improving Learning and Motivation through Educational Games: Multidisciplinary Approaches*, IGI Global, 2011.

[28] J. Janssen, O. Verschuren, D. Levac, J. Ermers and M. Ketelaar, "Structured game-related group therapy for an adolescent with Acquired Brain Injury: A case report," *Journal of pediatric rehabilitation medicine,* no. 5.2, pp. 125-132, 2012.

[29] B. Herbelin, J. Ciger and A. L. Brooks, "Customising games for non-formal rehabilitation," *International Journal on Disability and Human Development ,* no. 10.1, pp. 5-9, 2011.

Development of Exergame-based Virtual Trainer for Physical Therapy using Kinect

Baihua Li, Mark Maxwell, Daniel Leightley, Angela Lindsay*, Wendy Johnson*, Andrew Ruck**

Manchester Metropolitan University (b.li@mmu.ac.uk)
* NHS Lothian, ** Consard Limited

Abstract. We present the development of a virtual trainer for use by physio-therapists and patients in exercise based physiotherapy programmes. It allows a therapist to tailor exercise requirements to the specific needs and challenges of individual patients. Patients can select different programmes and follow a coach avatar to perform recorded exercises based on their needs. The Microsoft Kinect has been implemented as a means to track user's body movements. This enables immersive and natural interaction between the user and virtual tuition world. Most importantly, the recorded skeletal joint data facilitates quantitative analysis and feedback of patient's body movements. The proof of concept has been implemented and tested by 15 volunteers. Preliminary study shows the potential of using Kinect as a low cost solution for virtual physiotherapy training at home or clinic settings.

Keywords: Virtual physiotherapy, serious games, Kinect, rehabilitation.

1   Introduction

Rehabilitation programmes involving physical exercise and assistance with carrying out daily living tasks are undertaken by patients recovering from serious medical conditions, such as stroke, brain or physical injury. Supervised physio-therapy or occupational therapy start before discharge from hospital and continue when the patient returns home. Such clinic based approaches are expensive for the health service to provide. Numerous barriers (e.g. physical, economic, social and psychological factors) have been identified which prevent people from regularly participating. In view of increasing demand for healthcare services and modernisation of healthcare provision, there is an urgent need for the health-care system to make use of technological advances to deliver a more accessible and cheaper alternative to conventional physiotherapy and occupational therapy [12].

A lack of motivation has been identified as a major problem in therapy sessions, often caused by the repetitive nature of exercises [2]. Computer games have shown the potential to improve patients' adherence in rehabilitation [3]. Investigations have been carried out into the use of interactive multimedia and off-the-shelf games for physical rehabilitation [11, 12]. It was found that whilst positive results were present, various issues were identified. A main problem is that many games were not designed with rehabilitation in mind, therefore they do not specifically target the problems that patients have. Off-the-shelf games could actually cause frustration and anger in the person undergoing rehabilitation due to the fact that the gameplay can be too difficult and not adjustable to suit individual situations.

We aim to develop a low-cost virtual training computer application for patients who need to undertake regular physical exercise or cognitive tasks at home. It will enable people to follow a course of personalised rehabilitation exercises. The design of the virtual trainer will adapt to individual needs, differences and progress of user's therapy regime. State of the art motion sensing device Kinect is employed as a means of capturing player's movements, ultimately allowing for gestures and movements to become the gameplay input and to be analysed quantitatively for feedback. The proof of concept game "Theraplay" has been developed and tested [1]. The clinical scenario we target is rehabilitation of elderly people, but the concept of design is applicable to other problems in physiotherapy or occupational therapy, such as stroke and injuries which can be improved by regular and targeted exercise.

2 Design for users experiencing age-related changes

2.1 Visual cueing

Older people are likely to suffer from some degree of visually impairment. Visual cues can significantly improve the performance of participants to perform movements. When walking along a path marked by lines or markers, participants took longer strides with each step as well as a quicker speed [12]. Though the exact cause for this improvement is not clear, the landmarks gave the user an idea of how far they are stepping. It has also been reported that using large musical symbols and mirroring user's movements visually on screen were much more appealing and encouraging in a dance game [2]. It is interesting to find that intuitive visual feedback of player's movements seems to be an effective way to engage the player.

2.2 Player-controller: natural interaction through body movement

It has been a concern that elderly or impaired people have trouble adjusting to the use of new technologies, especially any advanced functions [7]. It is important to keep them in their comfort zone and use something they are familiar with, since they already suffer from restriction due to their disability and age. Further restriction (e.g. performing exercises unaided, complex equipments and intrusive sensors) should be avoided [2, 8]. Although the Nintendo Wii is perceived to be a possible tool for use with the elderly due to its success with younger people, the Microsoft Kinect does not require any form of a hand-held controllers or body worn sensors. The concept of using natural body movements and gestures of the player as gameplay controller is a new trend in exergaming, and a promising feature for people with physical, cognitive or age-related changes and impairments. Investigation of the suitability of the new technology for rehabilitation has been carried out, for example as demonstrated by the Rehabilitation Gaming System [4].

2.3 Design guidelines

Guidelines were stated by Gerling et al. [7] for the creation of a rehabilitation game for older users. One significant point made from these guidelines is that a bigger tolerance for gesture execution should be allowed rather than having to be very precise. Fatigue should be managed through pacing, as lack of stamina is typical of such a user group. Dynamically addressing difficulty was again brought up in this report. Simple gestures that map to real world manoeuvres are preferable in supporting gesture learning, as these people may have very limited or no experience with games.

It was found that more than 50% of the problems were due to usability related issues [6, 10]. In particular,

- learn-ability: how difficult it is to learn to use a device, to understand and to integrate functioning instruction.
- efficiency: the extent to which technological applications satisfy users's needs, avoiding frustration and dissatisfaction.
- memorability of device's functions: a measure of this can be obtained by considering the time needed to perform a previously experienced task.
- errors: how often the product can induce errors, and how easily it recovers from these errors.
- satisfaction: users' attitude and adoption of technological applications which could be influenced by the pleasure derived from their usage.

Considering the problems that come with old people, reducing the number of options, the speed of game elements and required reaction time could positively affect the demand for cognitive resources and information manipulation [5]. Guidelines for elderly entertainment should consider: therapy appropriate range of motion and focus diverted exercise matching with individual motor skills, meaningful tasks, appropriate cognitive challenges, simple objective and interface, motivational feedback, creation of new learning, and sensitivity to decreased sensory acuity and slower responses.

3 Implementation of virtual trainer Theraplay for physical therapy

Based on our study on design for elderly people, a imitation game, namely virtual trainer "Theraplay", was developed by making use of the prevailing Kinect technology. Such an application aims to provide an assistive tool for people who need to take regular physical exercise at home.

3.1 Motion tracking and gesture recording using Kinect

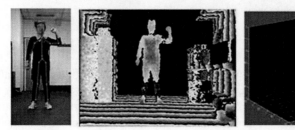

Fig. 1. Analysis of human movements from Kinect RGB, depth and skeleton images.

Microsoft Kinect has been widely used as the state of art motion tracking sensor in gaming. It is portable, easy to set up and allows operation in normal home or clinic settings. It records the body movements of the user in front of it at a speed of 30 frames per second (fps) for depth and colour stream in real-time. Field of view angle of Kinect can achieve 43 degrees vertical and 57 degrees horizontal. The vertical tilt range of the camera is +/- 27 degrees. The Kinect provides skeleton tracking for up to 6 people, of which 2 players can be active. As shown in Fig. 1, the skeleton of a user consists of key body parts presented by 20 anatomical joints with each joint providing a 3 dimensional x, y and z values. Each joint can be described as tracked or inferred. Inferring a joints requires estimating were the joint is likely to be based on the location of the other joints. The accuracy of 3D joint location is centimetre-level which is adequate for rehabilitation games and comparable with marker-based systems.

3.2 User play modes

The virtual trainer consists of two modes: physiotherapist mode and patient mode as shown in Fig. 2. In the physiotherapist mode, a physiotherapist can personally perform prescription movements and postures. These movements are recorded and can be played back through a 3D on-screen avatar, so that the physiotherapist can check and edit before storing them in an exercise database. This means in a therapist can record various movements and distribute them to patients according to individual needs. In the patient mode, a patient selects an exercise from the list of exercises. The selected exercise can be played back on a coach avatar. The user can preview the movement, know what to expect and then follow the coach to exercise themself. The user's exercise is captured by Kinect and displayed on the user's avatar during exercise.

Patients should try to copy the movement as accurately as they can, for example to keep in rhythm or pose similarity with the coach avatar. Tolerance is set to allow movements when are sufficiently close to the coach avatar, avoiding frustration. User performance and body postures are analysed. The patient gains a high score by correctly performing and completing the required exercises. Music and songs are used to create entertaining environment and improve user's performance.

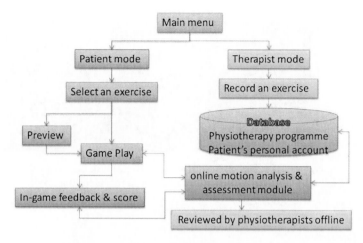

Fig. 2. Virtual trainer Theraplay structure chart

3.3 Interface

The interface design of Theraplay is shown in Fig. 3. Screens in each patient and therapist modes contain two avatars. One is linked to the patient/therapist (mirroring their movements in real-time); the other serves as a vessel to replay a pre-recorded movement. To avoid a cluttered screen and distract user attention, the avatar was rendered concisely using 14 joints. The depth image of Kinect is shown in the bottom right corner. It helps the user keep track the field of view and easily adjust the Kinect tilt angle by using "Change Kinect Angle" button provided on the interface.

Users should be able to use Theraplay on their own without requiring another person to assist with game control. However, if the user is out of range of the Kinect, skeletal joint data will be scrambled. To solve this problem, a countdown timer (e.g. 5 seconds) is implemented at the beginning of recording. This allows the user sufficient time to get into position after clicking the button to start Kinect. Meanwhile, Theraplay provides a trimming function that allows removal of any scrambled data at the end of recording before the data are saved.

Checkboxes of limbs was designed in the therapist mode. It allows the therapist to specify any body limb or combination of limbs for assessment. When replaying on the coach avatar, body limbs relevant to the exercise are displayed in blue, distinguishing with the colour used for other body parts.

We have attempted to use hand gestures (e.g. pushing and waving) to begin or stop data recording or gameplay. The results from testing were unsatisfying. This is because the command gestures may not be always detected properly. When performing exercises including gestures similar to those command gestures, the game will work inappropriately. People with cognitive or physical difficulties could find it even more difficult and frustrating to use gestures to control the game.

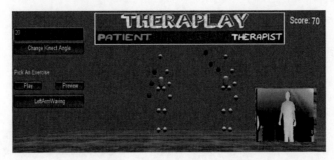

Fig. 3. Theraplay interface. The arm of coach avatar (right) is in blue, indicating relevant body part to the exercise. The arm of user's avatar (left) is in red, indicating incorrect movements. This turns to green when correct.

3.4 Feedback

Due to the varying ability from patient to patient, a successful game requires the ability to adapt to users' motor skill level [10]. The challenge and feeling of self-improvement is what motivates the patient to continue exercising. The user will need to be prompted when they are doing something wrong, but also given the correct indication to allow them to fix or improve their movement so that they will benefit from playing the game. This feature also means that as a patient improves, they do not outgrow the usefulness of the game as it will adapt to their improvements, providing an ever-increasing challenge.

In Theraplay, a in-game score is provided on screen. This will increase continuously while the patient's movement is within the acceptable range of accuracy as the coach avatar replays the movement. The score can then be used as a reference point to show how well the patient did compared with their previous performance. An important feature of Theraplay is direct visual feedback on user's movement presented on user's avatar during exercise. The patient will not have to check the score as the only means of telling how well they performed. Different colours of the joints on the user avatar are used to indicate satisfaction to the player's movement. For example, green indicates good mimic inside of the accepted range, while red indicates that the patient is performing the movement incorrectly with the coach.

Joint data of the player are calculated and compared with the coach avatar to assess the quality of the exercise in terms of posture and rhythm. Tolerance on joint angles and timing is used to setup the acceptable range. We have developed machine learning based action recognition method to automatically identify if an exercise is performed correctly [9]. The average recognition accuracy can achieve 90% on 10 testing exercises.

3.5 System development architecture

Unity3D is a cross platform (e.g. Windows, Mac OS, Xbox and mobile) and powerful game engine that comes complete with an intuitive set of tools to create interactive 3D content. There are thousands of ready-made assets available and a vast knowledge sharing community. It is an ideal game engine allowing quick production of prototyping games for feasibility and concept proof.

Unity does not natively provide connectivity for the Kinect. Accessing the Kinect in Unity3D can be achieved using OpenNI/NITE or third-party plugin Zigfu. OpenNI/NITE requires both the OpenNI framework to be installed as well as the Primesense NITE middleware for integration of the Kinect into Unity. However, this framework and its installation could be deemed too complicated to our targeted user group. In our game design, we chose Microsoft SDK driver and used Zigfu to connect the Kinect into Unity. The developed game is standalone, it runs on Windows machine with Microsoft Kinect SDK installed. The architecture of the virtual trainer development is shown in Fig. 4

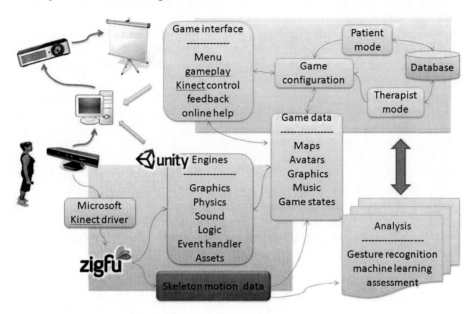

Fig. 4. Architecture of the Kinect-based virtual trainer development

4 Evaluation and testing

A range of excises at different difficulty levels have been recorded for testing. These include: 1) static posture matching, 2) simple uni-limb movements, 3) simple multi-limb movements and coordination, 4) complex uni-limb movements, such as changing route, speed matching, and combined postures, 5) complex multi-limb coordination, symmetry and asymmetry.

The prototype and recorded excises were evaluated by 15 volunteers of age from 18 to 65. Some of the subjects were specialists in physiotherapy and computing in addition to the general user population. Therapists were able to provide suggestions about the system therapeutic's effect and functionality requirements in clinic settings. Computer specialists could give their opinion on more technical aspects, for example code optimisation, system design and robustness of posture assessment to individual variations. General users evaluated usability and system applicability, including system setup, interface, control, visual clarity and feedback.

We first explained and demonstrated the functions of the prototype system to the users undertaking testing. Then the user was required to explore every function and try out by him/herself. At the end they were required to complete a survey consisting of eleven questions. These questions can be split among three major aspects:

Therapeutic domain: 1) Do you feel the application was beneficial to your therapy? 2) Do you feel the display of movements on the virtual therapist helped you to correctly perform the movements? 3) Did you think the assessment was appropriate? 4) Do you think such system can be an alternative to face-to-face clinic-based interventions?

Welfare: 5) Did you feel that it is easy to setup the system including the Kinect? 6) Did you feel comfortable during the playing experience? 7) Did you find that it is easy to use and understand? 8) Would the imitation game improve your motivation to perform the exercises?

Engagement value: 9) Did you think visual display of player's movements and indication of correct/incorrect postures helped your engagement? 10)Did you feel challenged? 11) Did it feel fun?

Each question was scored into 5 levels from strongly agree (100%) to strongly disagree (0%). The results of evaluation from 15 subjects is shown in Fig.5. At the end of questionnaire, open text space was provided for suggestion on e.g. how you think the system could be improved. Main suggestions centred on adding variation in gameplay to increase fun and user adherence. Many users also think the assessment criteria could be relaxed, allowing variation when individuals take an exercise in a slightly different way.

5 Discussion

Active participation in rehabilitation programs increases the benefit and effectiveness of therapy [2]. In the current proof of concept design, the program fulfills a similar role in therapy as a virtual trainer. Patients are required to mimic the designed exercises. Although visual feedback and scoring on movement accuracy etc. show promise in helping patient's engagement in short term, long-term patients motivation in rehabilitative context needs to be addressed. Preliminary studies on understanding motivational requirements in doing rehabilitative exercises show many factors that can influence on the patients level of motivation, such as social functioning, patient-therapist relationship, goal-setting, environment, meaningful rehabilitative tasks, recreational activities, positive feedback and music.

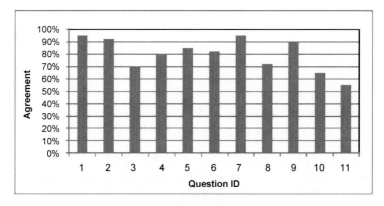

Fig. 5. Ratings of each question agreement in the evaluation questionnaire.

The prototype tool takes an imitation-based approach to monitor user performance. We have successfully developed real-time posture and movement assessment techniques that underpin the fundamentals of scoring. This provides a robust underlying framework to further develop the prototype into a fully-fledged game. In order to achieve this end, we envisage the inclusion of motivation-driven game context, contents and gameplay.

6   Conclusion

The imitation-based virtual trainer [1] could provide an assistive tool as an alternative to traditional face-to-face clinic-based interventions, reducing the need for clinic visits. We proposed the use of Kinect technology, enabling full body movements to become the gameplay input and to be analysed quantitatively for feedback. Such techniques underpin the development of complex exergames that encourage patients' engagement with their physiotherapy regimes. We have found that helping users feel motivated and engaged through motivational, recreational activities was crucial to the success of using such technology. Developing motivation-driven functional games with appealing gameplay would be a major focus to improve the current design.

Machine intelligence will be further explored for quantitative assessment on the similarity and variation of postures and kinematics. Abnormal and risky movements (e.g. risk of fall) could also be a focus of detection, so as to automatically generate risk alerts. Novel methods need to be investigated to interpret high volume data inputs from the sensor, and also possibly inputs from cognitive assessment and medical conditions. By mapping these onto patient profiles, low volume summary can be created for the supervising therapist. Such machine intelligence would be novel and advance to many general exercise/sports games.

Acknowledgments. This project is supported by MMU Knowledge Exchange and Innovation Fund. We would like to thank project partners NHS Lothian and Consard Limited for their support and constructive clinical advice.

References

[1] Theraplay video demo. www.youtube.com/watch?v=VorEbWMf2fE

[2] Arntzen, A.: Game based learning to enhance cognitive and physical capabilities of elderly people: concepts and requirements. Engineering and Technology 60, 63–67 (2011)

[3] Cameirão, M.S., Bermúdez, I.B.S., Duarte Oller, E., Verschure, P.F.: The rehabilitation gaming system: a review. Stud Health Technol Inform 145, 65–83 (2009)

[4] Cameirão, M.S., I Badia, S.B., Oller, E.D., Verschure, P.F.: Stroke rehabilitation using the rehabilitation gaming system (RGS): initial results of a clinical study. Annual Review of CyberTherapy and Telemedicine (2008)

[5] Flores, E., Tobon, G., Cavallaro, E., Cavallaro, F.I., Perry, J.C., Keller, T.: Improving patient motivation in game development for motor deficit rehabilitation. In: Int. Conf. Advances in Computer Entertainment Technology. pp. 381–384 (2008)

[6] Gamberini, L., Raya, M.A., Barresi, G., Fabregat, M., Ibanez, F., Prontu, L.: Cognition, technology and games for the elderly: An introduction to ELDER-GAMES project. PsychNology Journal 4(3), 285–308 (2006)

[7] Gerling, K., Livingston, I., Nacke, L., Mandryk, R.: Full-body motion-based game interaction for older adults. In: ACM Conf. Human Factors in Computing Systems (2012)

[8] Koyanagi, K., Fujii, Y., Furusho, J.: Development of VR-STEF system with force display glove system. In: Int. Conf. Augmented Tele-existence (2005)

[9] Leightley, D., Darby, J., Li, B., McPhee, J.S., Yap, M.H.: Human activity recognition for physical rehabilitation. In: IEEE Int. Conf. Systems, Man, and Cybernetics. pp. 261–266 (2013)

[10] Omelina, L., Jansen, B., Bonnechere, B., Van Sint Jan, S., Cornelis, J.: Serious games for physical rehabilitation: designing highly configurable and adaptable games. In: Int. Conf. Disability, Virutal Reality & Associated Technologies. pp. 195–201 (2012)

[11] Rego, P., Moreira, P.M., Reis, L.P.: Serious games for rehabilitation: A survey and a classification towards a taxonomy. In: IEEE Int. Conf. Sys. Tech. (2010)

[12] Vuong, C.H., Ingalls, T., Abbas, J.J.: Transforming clinical rehabilitation into interactive multimedia. In: ACM Int. Conf. Multimedia. pp. 937–940 (2011)

Digital Game Aesthetics of the iStoppFalls Exergame

Hannah R. Marston[1], Michael Kroll[1], Dennis Fink[1] and Sabine Eichberg[1]

[1]Institute of Movement and Sport Gerontology, German Sport University Cologne
{h.marston@dshs-koeln.de/marstonhannah@hotmail.com,
m.kroll@dshs-koeln.de,
D.Fink@dshs-koeln.de, Eichberg@dshs-koeln.de}

Abstract. The objective of this paper is to provide an overview of the iS-toppFalls exergames, in association with digital game genres and aesthetics. This paper aims to present the links between game theory and the developed exergames presented in this paper, resulting in a series of proposed recommendations. Although there is a growing body of work associated to exergames and health rehabilitation there is little work focusing and identifying game theory and exergames. For the future development of exergames a series of proposed recommendations have been suggested to facilitate researchers, practitioners and participants in gaining further understanding of the use of exergames for health rehabilitation in particular, fall prevention. To the knowledge of the authors, the iStoppFalls is the first ambient assisted exercise program (AAEP) which utilizes 21st Century digital game technology with a primary focus on fall prevention.

Keywords: Rehabilitation, Fall Prevention, Perceptual Opportunities, Digital Games

1   Introduction

Life expectancy across Europe is set to increase and the statistics indicate this population explosion is not going to slow down in the coming decades. It is estimated by 2020, the European population will increase from 894 million to 910 million people, and this is especially prevalent for populations aged 85 years and older. It is anticipated the age of the population from 2020 will be 14 million people which will rise to 40 million by 2050 [1].

Amongst ageing cohorts, the experience of falls is a common occurrence, due to the decrease of strength and balance, to changes in gait, falls can be experienced indoors, via tripping over rugs or outdoors whilst walking to and from the garden. Digital game technologies have been utilized in recent years for the purpose of health rehabilitation [see 2]. The utilization and implementation of such technologies may aid older adults to conduct regular physical activity in the comfort of their home resulting in a decrease of the risk of falling. An example is the iStoppFalls system which has been designed and developed to facilitate physical activity amongst adults aged 65+ years. Exergaming is relatively new and has become a fashionable area of games and health research since the release of the Nintendo™ Wii console (2005). It is suggested that there is a potential for exergaming to facilitate physical activity as a means of delivering home based exercises offering several positive elements to prospective users focusing on compliance and adherence to exercise:

- Utilization of exergames have the benefit to engage users of all ages but in particular older adults in physical activity which in turn has the potential to reduce fall risk;
- They may ensure higher compliance with exercise intervention than complete standard exercise interventions;
- Exercise within the home offers the possibility for older adults to engage in innovative forms of exercise than with conventional options (gym class or community based exercise programs); they provide a way of tracking exercise compliance over time; and have the potential to provide encouragement and motivation, if compliance starts to fail.

Exergames have the ability to provide users with a competitive environment leading to the experience of engagement and fun. The notion of exercise, coupled with gaming may have the advantage to motivate persons to complete the required exercises, whilst positively engaging with the virtual environment (VE). With the influx of academic interest associated to gaming and health there has been various studies utilizing the Sony Play Station® (PS) Eyetoy as a means of interaction via gesture to assess the feasibility of this technology for similar purposes. Earlier studies have sought to design and develop purpose built hard/software for the same objectives [see 2]. More recently the Microsoft™ Kinect console (2010) can facilitate users to interact with digital games through gesture and speech recognition without the need of a game pad or remote. To date there is little published research within the health and gerontology fields focusing on the utilization of the Kinect console, with the exception of iStoppFalls.

Little work has focused on the aesthetics and game theory being implemented into exergames and purpose built technologies aimed at prospective health benefits towards older users. However, one study designed and developed the PlayFit system by [3] aimed at reducing sedentary behavior amongst teenagers. The aims of this paper are: (1) to provide an overview of digital game aesthetics theory, (2) identify and discuss the aesthetics which have been exploited in the iStoppFalls project, and (3) propose a series of recommendations to develop this work further for future exploitation amongst users of the iStoppFalls system and general exergames.

2 Defining Digital Games

Genres can be associated with a variety of entertainment mediums, for example: literature, films, television programs and digital games [4]. Several researchers [4-12] have attempted to define the term game genre to aid a greater insight for researchers and consumers, taking into account the classification of digital games to facilitate consumers with suitable information based upon age and content descriptors. Marston and McClenaghen [13] have attempted to provide a greater understanding of the exergame genre reviewing previous taxonomies created by [4], who aimed to identify genres via activities performed within games. Mueller et al. [7] integrated game elements into four groups (Parallel/Non-parallel', 'Competitive/Non-Competitive', 'Exertion/Non-Exertion and Combat/Non-Combat) and focuses on user's perspectives rather than hardware. Adams [8-9] suggests there are more facets associated to the categorization of genre including: setting, audience, theme and purpose. Further [8-9] contends that games are determined by gameplay, including the challenges faced by gamers and performing the necessary actions to complete the challenge of task. Oh & Lang [10] constructed a matrix comprising of terms associated (e.g. exertainment, dance simulation and physical gaming) from 23 articles and the most popular term was exergaming. Lindley [11] uses a classification pane initially 2-D utilizing ludology, narratology and simulation. However, a 3-D plane is introduced by adding gambling to the plane in addition to fiction/non-fiction and virtual/physical. Swayer & Smith [12] taxonomy takes a different standpoint whereby genre (education, advergames, and games for health) and sector (government, defense, healthcare, and corporate) are primarily considered.

Prospective recommendations by [13] included: game analysis of online and off-the-shelf games to identify exact game elements; establish serious game guidelines to aid clinicians/ users', consider and revise the current classification systems and implement a games for health classification system to facilitate clinicians and users with suitable software, execute longitudinal studies to gain in-depth understanding of utilizing game software for rehabilitation and finally, identify a constructive methodology, to assist with a suitable taxonomy for all sectors.

3   Digital Game Aesthetics

Many digital games incorporate or illuminate aesthetics to their players. Murray [14] deems interactive digital environments (IDE's), such as games, to incorporate three elements. These may be individual or combined within one game:

- Immersion is experienced during play when a particular gamer experiences the feeling of being lost in the environment or story.
- Agency is described when control occurs by the gamer in the digital environment.
- Transformation is to feel or become someone else or something else which many gamers experience during play.

The aesthetics defined by [14] were taken from the properties of IDE's which include: (1) procedural which comprise of a set of rules and rule based descriptions of places, people and objects used by gamers during play. (2) Participatory is described by the break-up of the digital environment enabling the gamer to value and understand the pleasure(s) gained, (3) spatial is described as the portrait of a navigable space either in a game or digital format, for example a website, conversation or a 3-D environment, and (4) encyclopedic is the availability of digital environments offering the potential to deliver information which is too vast for the human mind. The experience of aesthetics does not provide an overall understanding to the meaning but can provide a positive notion of pleasure [4]. Therefore, in relation to the emergence of a new digital medium, Murray [15] presents three stages:

- "The embryonic medium – users participate in the new medium prior to the technology itself being available to support it;
- The incunabula medium – is available in part at least, but users are still learning how to specifically create for the medium and;
- The fully fledge medium – new forms arise which are specific to the medium and make the most of its capabilities."

Murray [14] summarizes, the majority of VE's are in stage two (The incunabula medium), based upon the notion of not knowing exactly what the environments are trying to do. Alternatively, the formal abstract design tools (FADT) framework proposed by [15] comprises of: (1) intention, (2) perceivable consequence, and (3) story. In the following section, these three elements are explained:

Intention is the pleasure experienced by the user while understanding the purpose of the game and deciding what the subsequent action(s) should be to progress onto the next level. Perceivable consequence and agency are similar within gaming. Users experience the pleasure of agency through the intent of actions and the perceivable consequence(s) of the actions during play. For many in the gaming community, story is obvious. However, there may be countless stories, or a background story, which provides an insight into the quest (if it is an adventure game), but for some as [4] suggest, games like Tetris, actually do not have a story or narrative. Therefore, users have the opportunity to create their own story through play. Moreover, some could argue when play has ceased, a story has been formed from the player; the player is telling the story to a friend based on their success.

Exploration of perceptual opportunities (PO) has been undertaken by [4]. PO's are items comprising of a role within digital content exhibited via game play. The approach to designing and understanding the inter-relationships of PO's is known as perceptual modeling. A modeling technique can aid the understanding of the PO relationships within larger structures or environments, in particular, a digital game and has the possibility to represent game play overtime. A PO map [4] illustrates the relationship of attributes found within a game environment and their structures which configure these inter-relationships. Each attribute and sub-group will be explained in the proceeding section.

3.1 Understanding Perceptual Opportunities (PO)

Fencott et al. [4] explains; sureties are everyday details which are predictable within the environment. This type of detail can be identified through elements such as lamp posts or incidental items. The real world is generally a chaotic world and this can be followed through into a VE. Furthermore, sound can be implemented to add to the atmospheric ambience of the VE during game play.

Surprises are used in an environment to provide an emphasis [16] and to precipitate conscious learning. The inclusion of surprises is to deliver a purpose and to accumulate users providing an experience. This facet can be implausible but beneficial to the environment however, they can be plausible but unexpected. There are three basic types (1) attractors, (2) connectors and (3) rewards [4].

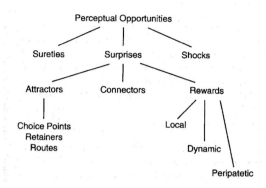

Figure 1: PO Map and contributing attributes [4]

Attractors are used to draw the attention of a gamer to a particular object. They can be seen or heard and can be mysterious, active, sensational and complex. Choice points are associated with attractors and provide a choice of alternative goals for the same attractor. Retainers; are a group of surprises that constitute sites of interest to the user, which may include interaction, and seek to provide the purpose of the VE. Routes can be implicit or explicit, drawing visitors around the VE which aim to display all important content. Surprises can also have connectors; which assist in the satisfaction of goals in response to the attractors via four facets: (a) basic interaction technologies, (b) information objects (maps or signposts), (c) online assistance and (d) the degrading of reality, the removal of detail to deflect visitors back to areas of interests. Rewards; can be various including local, peripatetic and dynamic, and they can deliver a specific memorable experience and ensure visitors linger in a certain area from time to time [4].

The iStoppFalls project comprises of several technologies and interfaces to facilitate the users with physical activity including educational material, three exergames and a social networking component via Google TV. For the purpose of this paper, the authors will focus on the exergame aspect, comprising of three different variations of one game to facilitate with the balance training taking into account the principles of the Otago program [17], these are: Hills 'n' Skills, the Bumble Bee Park and The Bistro.

3.2 iStoppFalls Exergame Components

Three key points were ascertained for training balance skills and comprised of (1) weight shifting (2) knee bending and (3) stepping. One or more of the different key points were implemented into the three games whereby, the level of difficulty is increased and the following points were reviewed for inclusion into each game:

- Reduce upper limb support (a chair as option for upper limb support is provided);
- Reduce base of feet support;
- Include arms (for example reaching); and

- Combine the three key point's weight shifting, knee bending and stepping step by step.
- Include dual tasks to shift or divide attention

Across all three games, the user is shown a series of icons situated on the screen (c.f. Figure 2). The 'Kinect tracked 100%' icon displays to the user their stance at that point in time and is located at the bottom left hand side of the screen. At the bottom right hand side of the screen, there is an icon displaying 'Level, Points and Progress' which informs the user of his/her progress. Situated along the bottom of the screen, the words 'Pause, Instructions, and Abort' are shown allowing users to engage and recap with the VE at their convenience Finally, the icon 'SMM not recording' informs the user that their senior mobility monitor (SMM) is not collecting data. However, this would change to SMM is recording, if the SMM is connected which it is when the participants are undertaking their training schedule.

A series of dual tasks have been implemented into the later levels of Games 1 and 2. One of the dual-tasks is a series of mathematical equations (subtraction and addition) where an equation is displayed to the user via the screen. The user is required to choose the correct answer from four options, by raising their left or right hand. Additional dual tasks are implemented into the games, which require participants to count birdhouses, and memorize objects. As the level of difficulty increases so do the tasks. For example, the first task is to memorize three objects, than four etc.). The level of difficulty also increases for the mathematical equations, for example; single-digits will be displayed followed by double digits (e.g. 4+5; 22-13). Finally, coins have been implemented into the game levels, which users can collect as they travel around the circuits. If a user collects a coin, they are rewarded with points.

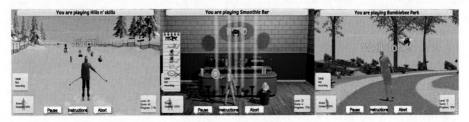

Fig. 2: iStoppFalls exergame interfaces

3.2.1   Game 1 – Hills 'n' Skills

The purpose of the game is to solve a slalom course, the user receive points for time, passed gates, and additional tasks. To start the game, the user is required to stand up straight in front of the Kinect and to pay attention to the automatic countdown. If they need to avoid an obstacle then they lean their body to the left or right side. Snowmen have been implemented as additional obstacles. Points are rewarded by correctly passing a gate but no points are rewarded or deducted if they collide with a snowman. A total of 51 levels have been developed and implemented into the Hills 'n' Skills game. The level of difficulty is increased after level 17 by reducing the spaces between the gates as the participant is demanded to shift his/her weight more often.

3.2.2   Game 3 – Bumble Bee Park

The purpose of Game 3 is to walk through a park and avoid bees. There are 45 levels in the Bumble Bee game, which allows to increase the level of difficulty reducing the lower limb support by starting with a low step and finish on a high step in the higher levels. The initial game interface illustrates several facets of interest to the user: which are different to the common elements explained above. The main element is the path which the user 'walk/step' along to complete the level. Coins are placed around the footpath, which the user has to collect and avoid the bumble bees coming towards the avatar. Dual tasks have been implemented into this game, and follow a similar process as previously explained.

3.2.3   Game 2 – The Bistro

The objective of The Bistro game is to collect a series of ingredients to make a sandwich or a smoothie. The primary focus of movement is to either step or to lean and shift the body weight to the left or right side. There are a total of 22 levels. Initially, the user is required to collect all of the ingredients which are falling from the ceiling. As the user progresses through the levels, a recipe list is displayed showing the user the exact ingredients needed to complete the recipe. The ingredients are collected by the user leaning or stepping to the left or right and collecting the specific ingredient into the bowl. If the user collects all of the correct items in the correct order, a tick is shown at the side of the word and the 'green button' which enables the user to 'make the smoothie.' If the user is unable to collect a certain ingredient, then a red cross is displayed at the side of the item. A spider has been implemented into the game which appears intermittingly. The user is expected to avoid the spider, whilst collecting the ingredients. If the user does not avoid the spider or is unable to collect the items, they are thrown into the rubbish bin. A cookie has been implemented, enabling users to gain extra points if it is collected into their bowl.

3.3   Aesthetics of the iStoppFalls Exergame

In the following section the aesthetics of the exergame are identified and explained. Sureties: throughout all three games, the VE has been built to reflect a real setting for example, in Game 1 the types of sureties identified are rocks, trees, snow/men, gates, firs, and a finishing post. In Game 2, users can see trees, flowers, and natural foliage. Game 3 displays a typical coffee counter comprising of equipment (e.g. coffee maker), seating and signage found in a café.

Shocks: have been implemented to facilitate the execution of exercise but to add a sense of engagement within the VE. Additionally, in Game 1, users will experience the appearance of snowmen, appearing at different levels of the game, and in Games 2 and 3 bees and spiders appear intermittently. This makes the user lean to the right or left to avoid the animal and continue with the game objectives.

Surprises: can be found throughout all of the games, resulting in additional tasks (e.g. mathematical equations, memory tasks), while executing a stepping motion, bending or leaning exercise. Attractors: can be found immediately in Games 1 and 2, by following a certain path to complete the task. In Game 2, once the user has completed reading the instructions, by executing the stepping motion, the user will understand the avatar will 'walk' around the path. Additional attractors include coins, memory items (e.g. bird houses), and in addition to Game 1; snowmen, and gates. In Game 3 there is the recipe which the user has to follow and collect the correct items listed.

Choice points: are particularly noticeable in Game 1. While the user is skiing down the mountain, they are aware that they need to avoid the snowmen, ski through the gates (to gain points), collect the coins, complete the dual-task questions and reach the finish line. Routes: are simple across the three games. In Game 2, there is one primary route which is the path. Game 1, is the mountain hill, associated with the placing of gates/snowmen to form the 'route' and in Game 3, the user is expected to step or lean the length of the counter. Connectors: throughout Games 1-3, show a variety of detail to provide a sense of realism to the user within the VE. However, because of the game objectives each VE is not overloaded with connectors. There are several icons which provide the user with further information associated with their exercises, game level(s) and points. There are additional buttons accessible to the user placed at the bottom of the screen in the centre of the screen (Pause, Instruction and Abort). These buttons facilitate the user to choose their actions within the game or gain further information if they require a re-cap of a particular exercise. Rewards: are gained by the user by collecting coins, selecting the correct mathematical answer, or choosing the correct item or colour. Additional points are rewarded if the user completes the paths in the Bumble Bee game quicker, or in the Hills 'n' Skills game, if they bend their knees they will ski quicker resulting in further points. And in the Bistro game, if the cookie is caught points are added. Points are deducted if the user does not select the correct answer.

3.4 Aesthetic Framework – Murray (1997)

The aesthetics associated to the iStoppFalls exergame defined by [14] are procedural, based upon a specific set of algorithms implemented into the system which result in a set of rules being completed by the target audience (adults aged 65+ years) to complete the task. However, taking into account the work by [18], procedural rhetoric encompasses processes, logic and system rules, which [18] suggests, can shape persuasion and expression. One may think that the work by [18] could be integrated into the iStoppFalls exergame, based upon the example within the political section, which [18] claims can teach one about the political process through procedural rhetoric. However, it was never the intention to teach users about fall prevention directly through the iStoppFalls exergame, although educational material is provided to participants about fall prevention. Therefore, from this point onwards we will stick with the aesthetics of [14]. In Game 1, the user is expected to ski down the mountain, whilst avoiding snowmen, and going through the designated gates while collecting coins, answering mathematical equations, counting a certain number of objects in a specific colour and complete the question with the correct answer. In Game 2, the user has to walk around the path in the park avoiding bees, and executing dual-task exercises. In Game 3 depending upon the level of the game, the user is expected to collect all of the falling ingredients or in the later levels, collect a select number of ingredients as shown on the recipe list. As explained by [14], the emergence of new digital mediums the exergames can be categorized as stage 2 the incunabula medium. For example, designers and developers have the knowledge and skills to produce an exergame, yet there is still further knowledge needed to fully understand what is required of an exergame specifically aimed at a health benefit such as fall prevention.

3.5   Aesthetic Framework – Church (1999) - FADT's.

With regards to [15] aesthetics; story is relevant in so much as; the user is provided with the information to complete the circuit in Games 1 and 2 while avoiding obstacles through a series of exercises within a specified time limit. Users may create their own story relevant to their exercise program. For example; as users progress through the different levels, they may choose to tell and demonstrate to their friends, family and the research team. With this notion, it is suggested, a user could create their own story, of their game experiences as [4] proposed with Tetris. Intention can be identified by users, who experience the pleasure of the game while understanding the objectives of the environment. This is particularly relevant when associated to activities of daily living (ADL). For example; the participants in the real world are familiar with a park, restaurant, and sporting events. Finally, perceivable consequence may be experienced by users who are required to physically interact with the environment through body movement. All games require users to physically interact with the environment to complete and progress from one level to the next. Previously, interaction has been related to user's motion while holding a traditional game pad. However, there is no such technology in this project and therefore, physical movement by the user's body to initiate game interaction is required.

4   Recommendations for Future Work based on Exergames

The authors propose a series of recommendations which have been categorized into themes and it is anticipated these recommendations could provide designers, developers and users the ability to gain full capability from exergames which have a fall prevention focus:
Safety

- The ability to have additional support such as a chair for users who are categorized as frail. This would maintain a safety support;
- Individualized program and progression to avoid under- or overexertion

Interface of the Exergame

- All instructions should be clear and concise;
- Icons depicting the level, user progress and the type of course should be easily recognizable, and understandable;
- All icons should be easily recognizable and the use of voice recognition should be suitably implemented for users to be able to access this function;

Design of the Exergame

- All instructions should be clear and concise;
- No unnecessary features (colors, music, information) which distract the attention of the user from the basic intention/task/information;
- Implementing video to illustrate exercises should contain a series of instructions, the inclusion of suitable models and visual representation should be clearly defined;
- Gaining user feedback throughout the design and development is necessary to maintain suitable information for the final deployment;
- Consider and analyze videogame theory constructed by Bogost which could enable further design and developments associated to procedural rhetoric.

User motivation and engagement

- Integrate suitable leaning and bending exercises for all users (frail and active) providing an individualized program and progression for training;
- Positive and motivating feedback should be implemented to maintain user engagement;
- If the user executes a move that they shouldn't, (e.g. bumping into a snowman) points should not be given. However, points should also not be deducted to maintain motivation and engagement;
- Implementing dual tasks should be suitable for the level of the game, enabling the user to complete the questions sufficiently. Dual tasks should not be placed between obstacles such as snowmen and gates (Hills 'n' Skills game) which could result in a practical problem of reaching the answer sufficiently within the given time period. Therefore, dual tasks should appear at suitable distances throughout each level.
- Game challenges should facilitate user motivation resulting in completion of the exercise;
- Game difficulty should be steadily increased as the user progress through each level. Initially, if it is too difficult, this may prevent users from continuing their exercise program;

Study Execution

- Qualitative data collection is crucial to gain additional information from the users. Data collection could be in the form of one-to-one interviews and/or focus groups. The type of data collection which researchers could consider is:

— Users experiences during the study;
— Users challenges to using the technology;
— Elements of the game to be considered for a future re-design; and
— Take up of digital game play which has a health and physical fitness focus based upon the game development.

Choosing the correct quantitative approaches is crucial for such studies. There are a variety of physical and cognitive tests which can be utilized to assess fall prediction. If a future multi-centred study was to be conducted, researchers and clinicians need to discuss and agree upon a set of assessment tests which can be transferable into multiple languages and executed sufficiently.

5 Conclusions

To summarize, this paper has presented the theory of game aesthetics in conjunction with a purpose built AAEP to facilitate fall prevention aimed at adults 65+ years. This paper has shown based upon [14,15] theories have been implemented. In conjunction with the proposed recommendations, it is suggested these recommendations may facilitate researchers and developers to design and develop suitable exergames, primarily associated to fall prevention. Further, by taking into account the recommendations, this may assist users to engage more with purpose built AAEP's which would result in individual health benefits. Additional work is needed in the area of exergames and game theory to gain in-depth understanding of this phenomenon, especially in regards to health and fall prevention, which could facilitate design, development, execution of future studies and enable adherence and user engagement.

6 References

[1] World Health Organization, The "Demographic trends, statistics and data on ageing," Retrieved September 15, 2013, from, http://www.euro.who.int/en/ what-we-do/health-topics/Life-stages/healthy-ageing/data-and-statistics/ demographic-trends,-statistics-and-data-on-ageing

[2] Marston, H. R., & Smith, S. T. (2012). Interactive Videogame Technologies to Support Independence in the Elderly: A Narrative Review, Games for Health Journal: Research, Development, and Clinical Application, vol 1, no. 2: 139-159 DOI: 10.1089/g4h.2011.0008.

[3] Sluis-Thiescheffer, R. J. W., Tieben, R., Sturm, M. M., Schouten, B. (2013). An Active Lifestyle for Youths through Ambient Persuasive Technology. Implementing Activating Concepts in a School Environment. In B. Schouten, S. Fedtke, T. Bekker, M. Schijven & A. Gekker (Eds.), Conference Paper: *Games for Health: Proceedings of the 3rd european conference on gaming and playful interaction in health care, (pp. 293-308).* Wiesbaden: Springer Vieweg.

[4] Fencott, C., Lockyer, M., Clay, J., & Massey, P. (2012). Game Invaders, The Theory and Understanding of Computer Games. Hoboken, New Jersey, John Wiley & Sons, Inc.

[5] Botte, B., Matera, C., & Sponsiello, M. (2009). Serious Games between simulation and game. A proposal of taxonomy. Journal of e-Learning and Knowledge Society. 5(2), 11-21.

[6] Kickmeier-Rust, M. D (n.d) Talking Digital Educational Games. Retrieved August 8, 2013, from http://www.eightydays.eu/Paper/01%20Graz%20 Workshop.pdfAdams, E. (2009a). Fundamentals of Game Design. 2nd Edition, New Riders, Berkeley, CA, USA.

[7] Mueller, F., Gibbs, M. R., & Vetere, F. (2010). Taxonomy of Exertion Games. In Proceedings OZCHI 2008, December 8-12, 2008, Cairns, QLD, Australia, 2008.

[8] Marston, H. R., & McClenaghan, P. (2013). Play yourself fit: Exercise + Video games = Exergames, In K. Bredl and W. Bösche (Eds.), Serious Games and Virtual Worlds in Education, Professional Development, and Healthcare. Hershey, PA: Information Science Reference.

[9] Adams, E. (2009b). The Designer's Notebook: Sorting Out the Genre Muddle. July 9 2009. Gamasutra. Retrieved September 3, 2013, from http://www. gamasutra.com/view/feature/4074/the_designers_notebook_sorting_.php.

[10] Adams, E. (2009a). *Fundamentals of game design* (2nd ed.). Berkeley, CA: New Riders.

[11] Oh, Y., & Yang, S. Defining Exergames and Exergaming, In proceedings Meaningful Play Conference Paper, Michigan State University, East Lansing, Michigan, Retrieved April 7, 2012 from, http://meaningfulplay.msu.edu/ proceedings2010/mp2010_paper_63.pdf.

[12] Lindley, C. (2003). Game Taxonomies: A High Level Framework for Game Analysis and Design. Retrieved April 6 2012, from, http://www.gamasutra. com/view/feature/131205/game_taxonomies_a_high_level_.php?page=2. Gamasutra.

[13] Sawyer, B., & Smith, P. (2008). Serious Games Taxonomy. Presented at the Game Developers Conference 2008. Retrieved September 10, 2012. From http://www.dmill.com/presentations/serious-games-taxonomy-2008.pdf

[14] Murray, J. H. (1997). Hamlet on the Holodeck: The Future of Narrative in Cyberspace. New York: Free Press

[15] Church, D. (1999). Formal Abstract Design Tools. Featured in Gamasutra, July 16, 1999. Retrieved September 13 2013, from http://www.gamasutra. com/view/feature/3357/formal_abstract_design_tools.php.

[16] Whitelock, D., Brna, P., & Holland, S. (1996). What is the Value of Virtual Reality for Conceptual Learning? Towards a Theoretical Framework.

[17] Campbell. J. A., Robertson. M.C. (2003). Otago exercise program to prevent falls in older adults. Retrieved July 2012, from http://www.acc.co.nz/PRD_ EXT_CSMP/groups/external_providers/documents/publications_promotion/pr d_ctrb118334.pdf.

[18] Bogost, I. (2007). Persuasive Games: The Expressive Power of Videogames. MIT Press.

"Gabarello v.1.0" and "Gabarello v.2.0": Development of motivating rehabilitation games for robot-assisted locomotion therapy in childhood

Anna Lisa Martin[1], Ulrich Götz[1], Cornelius Müller[1], René Bauer[1]

[1]Zurich University of the Arts, Department of Design, Specialization in Game Design
{anna.martin, ulrich.goetz, cornelius.mueller, rené.bauer}@zhdk.ch

Abstract. Virtual rehabilitation games have the potential to increase children's motivation during robot-assisted locomotion therapy. Based on this approach, two target-group specific rehabilitation games were developed. „Gabarello v.1.0" and „Gabarello v.2.0" are controlled by the patient's motion in Hocoma's gait-driven orthosis Lokomat®, which provides biofeedback values of the patient's physical performance. These measurements are exploited to derive video game playability for the patient in real time. "Gabarello v.2.0" is connected to therapy devices through a specific middleware ("RehabConnex"). This set-up allows the extension of the game environment through the additional use of the sensor glove "PITS" (Institute of Neuroinformatics, ETH Zurich/University of Zurich) to complete a second task, while maintaining the game's key features. Both rehabilitation games turn therapy into a stimulating, self-motivated, fun experience, supporting both patients and therapists. This explorative approach might be used as guideline for future rehabilitation game developments.

Keywords: Rehabilitation games, robot-assisted locomotion therapy, motivation, Gabarello, RehabConnex, childhood

1 Introduction

Children's locomotive ability can be adversely affected by neurological disorders or injuries such as spinal cord injury, stroke or traumatic brain injury [1]. According to de Leon et al. [2], rehabilitation of patients with such injuries should include gait training. There is evidence that the desired function or movement has to be trained in a task-specific program [2]. Lünenburger et al. [1] report that robot-assisted gait therapy can increase the training duration and intensity for the patients while reducing the physical strain for the therapist. In attempting to optimize therapy and its sustainability, virtual reality (VR) scenarios can be integrated into rehabilitation to create a functional, purposeful and motivating context. VR is used as a therapeutic tool that provides assistance, immediate feedback, and real-time interactive experience [3]. The need for diversification, fun and motivation, particularly in pediatric rehabilitation, has been demonstrated in several investigations [e.g. 4]. The effect of VR can be enhanced if the interactive potential of video game scenarios is combined with therapeutic goals. The high level of evidence for using interactive computer games in motor rehabilitation of children was shown in various studies [e.g., 5].

Drawing from their experience designing games for therapeutic environments, game designers of the Zurich University of the Arts (ZHdK) in 2008 established an interdisciplinary collaboration with physicians, therapists and movement scientists (Rehab Research Group of the University Children's Hospital Zurich & Sensory Motor System Lab, ETH Zurich) to undertake the project "Gabarello v.1.0" (short for "Game Based Rehabilitation for Lokomat"). Following the successful implementation of "Gabarello v.1.0" [6], the development of meaningful therapeutic games was continued in the follow-up project "IMIC" (Innovative Movement Therapies in Childhood) from 2010 on [7]. "IMIC" aims to improve movement therapies for children with cerebral motor impairment using innovative, multi-task rehabilitation technologies for upper and lower extremities. "Gabarello v.2.0", was developed according to this extended strategy, and will be completed in 2014.

2 Development of "Gabarello v.1.0" & "Gabarello v.2.0"

The Rehabilitation Center for Children and Adolescents, Affoltern a. A. (University Children's Hospital Zurich) makes use of the gait-driven orthosis Lokomat® (Hocoma AG, Volketswil, Switzerland). In a stand-alone version of the gait robot, the motivation of a patient to participate actively in the locomotion therapy is primarily achieved through encouragement from a therapist. Both "Gabarello v.1.0" and "Gabarello v.2.0" are designed to support the therapist in maintaining the patient's motivation to complete therapeutic goals (Fig.1).

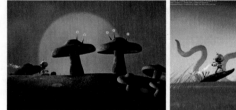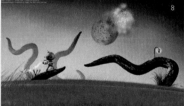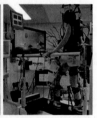

Fig. 1: Screenshots and settings of "Gabarello v.1.0" and "Gabarello v.2.0" (Source: ZHdK)

From the patient's point of view, the set-up of "Gabarello v.1.0" turns the Lokomat® from a physiotherapeutic tool into a full-body game controller. Patients influence the speed and abilities of a game character by the level of their active participation in the Lokomat® [8]. "Gabarello v.2.0" features "RehabConnex", a parallel "IMIC"-development, which serves as a middleware to connect a range of rehabilitation games with several rehabilitation devices ("Gabarello v.2.0" can be connected to the Lokomat® and the "Pediatric Interactive Therapy System" (PITS), developed by the Institute of Neuroinformatics, ETH Zurich and University of Zurich). The dual task "Gabarello v.2.0" aims to shift the patient's focus of attention from the gait locomotion to the upper extremities in order to further automate and improve gait training. During concept design and realization of the games, the experiences and recommendations of target group experts were the most important input. The observation and analysis of the therapist's tasks in gait-orthosis training situations led to first design paradigms. Later, target group specific requirements, needs and guidelines were evaluated, followed by the identification of possible game mechanics (e.g., system of rules and rewards, game usability, etc.). Several criteria were identified as paramount: (i) it was important that the games were self-explanatory for children as well as for therapists in order to avoid introducing additional stress to the therapy setting; (ii) the games had to be naturally, subtly and constantly motivating, even after several training sessions; (iii) they had to be gender-, and age-neutral; (iv) they had to be easily integrated into therapy and had not to distract the therapist from monitoring the patient and the software settings. The following description details specific similarities and differences of the two rehabilitation games:

In "Gabarello v.1.0" the patient controls the walking speed of an avatar through the detected level of the Lokomat®'s biofeedback, which is divided into three distinguished levels of effort. The avatar, an astronaut named "Nicolo", has landed on a dark planet. During "Nicolo's" circumnavigations of the planet he encounters lighting flowers (score items), setting them free on collision. "Nicolo" will need several circumnavigations of the planet on different rocky paths to reach all flowers.

"Gabarello v.2.0" is located on a distinct planet with obvious differences in vegetation, landscape and atmosphere. "Nicolo" encounters rose hips (score items) and aims at red clouds (score items) with his new feature, a rocket-enhanced backpack, which is triggered by the patient's opening and closing of the "PITS" glove. A hit at a red cloud results in rain, which leads to the immediate growth of more rose hips. Each time "Nicolo" has set a rose hip free, it is turned into a blue cloud. On the next circumvnavigation of the planet, the blue clouds will have turned into red clouds, providing new targets (score items) for "Nicolo's" rockets.

Both games define thresholds of the Lokomat®'s biofeedback, which can be manually adjusted to the patient's performance by the therapist. Depending on the patient's effort ("PlayerWalkState") the points awarded by each score item will vary between 1, 4 and 8. Each score item has initially 3 points, which are subtracted on collision with "Nicolo", according to the "PlayerWalkState". For "Gabarello v.1.0" the number of score items is finite and results in a maximal highscore; they are reduced over the elapsed training time. In "Gabarello v.2.0" the number of score items is infinite and is rebuilt over the course of gameplay; the final score depends on the overall gaming time elapsed. The two scoring mechanisms result in differences in gameplay motivation: "Gabarello v.1.0" makes the patient focus on the strategic choice of the avatar's paths to collect as many flowers as possible, whereas in "Gabarello v.2.0" the transformation of clouds into rose hips and vice versa guarantees a continuous motivation for scoring.

"Nicolo's" shape and abilities vary according to the current level of exertion of the patient. The visual feedback of the patient's effort is displayed through the changing length of "Nicolo's" legs and particle trails streaming from his backpack. The movement of "Nicolo's" legs can be synchronized to the walking rhythm of the Lokomat®. The level of exertion is directly linked to three different walking speeds of the avatar, which can enable the avatar to jump over obstacles and gaps.

The games take into account the types of trauma experienced by the patients, placing balanced demands upon physical and cognitive abilities during the gameplay and offering positive incentives only, even at minimal exertion. The level designs of both games feature modular "active" and "resting" phases. During "active" phases the patients need to react promptly to in-game events, while "resting" phases require less physical and cognitive effort. Even though the games differ in their graphic design, scoring system and control input, the modular level design is kept strictly comparable to provide a basis for future research on the outcome of single vs. dual task training.

The games use side-scrolling cameras to prevent the patient from typical coordination problems resulting from steering an avatar in the depth of perspective. The screen-zoom can be manually adjusted. The game graphics are kept deliberately simple, and offer both a high visual contrast in order to account for visual limitations of the patient, and ease-of-use by the therapist.

3 Outlook

"Gabarello v.1.0" was successfully integrated into the children's robot-assisted gait therapy at the Rehabilitation Center for Children and Adolescents. "Gabarello v.2.0" is currently being completed and will soon be ready for application. The game designers (ZHdK) will conduct exploratory research on both games, comparing the games with regard to gameplay experiences, measurable emotional responses and the physiological effort exerted through the active participation. The investigation should provide a conclusion on the functionality of the player-centered design in order to establish guidance for future meaningful therapeutic game developments.

References

[1] Lünenburger, L., Colombo, G., Riener, R.: Biofeedback for robotic gait rehabilitation. Journal of NeuroEngineering and Rehabilitation, 4(1), 1-11 (2007)

[2] de Leon, R.D., Hodgson, J.A., Roy, R.R., Edgerton, V.R.: Locomotor capacity attributable to step training versus spontaneous recovery after spinalization in adult cats. Journal of Neurophysiology, 79(3), 1329-1340 (1998)

[3] Bursting, A., Brown, R.: Virtual environments for real treatments. Polish Annals of Medicine, 17(10), 101-111 (2010)

[4] Brütsch, K. et al.: Virtual reality for enhancement of robot-assisted gait training in children with neurological gait disorders. Journal of Rehabilitation Medicine, 43(6), 493-499 (2011)

[5] Reid, D., Campbell K.: The use of virtual reality with children with cerebral palsy: a pilot randomized trial. Therapeutic Recreation Journal, 40(4), 255-68 (2006)

[6] Götz, U. et al.: A Virtual Reality System for Robot-Assisted Gait Training Based on Game Design Principles. Int. Conf. on Virtual Rehabil., pp. 1-2. IEEE (2011)

[7] Martin, A.L., Götz, U., Bauer, R.: IMIC - Innovative Movement Therapies in Childhood. In: Wiemeyer, J. (ed.) Serious in der Neurorehabilitation, Zeitschrift für Neurologie & Rehabilitation. Hippocampus, Bad Honnef (in press)

[8] Labruyère, R. et al.: Requirements for and impact of a serious game for neuro-pediatric robot-assisted gait training. Research in developmental disabilities, 34(11), 3906-3915 (2013)

Player-centred Design Model for psychophysiological adaptive Exergame Fitness Training for Children

Anna Lisa Martin[1] & Viktoria Jolanda Kluckner[1]

[1]Zurich University of the Arts, Department of Design, Specialization in Game Design
{anna.martin, viktoria.kluckner}@zhdk.ch

Abstract. Exergames are body-centered games, which are controlled by various physical activities. Since they are additionally motivating and cognitive demanding, they tend to be a beneficial alternative for holistic fitness training. Therefore, the exergame's design needs to guide the player in one's individual comfort and performance zone ("dual flow"). Thus, a real-time adaptive game-play must be provided by combining a pre-classification of the player's motor-skills and cognitive abilities, sensory-monitoring of psychophysiological player parameters while playing the game (e.g., heart rate, electroencephalogram, electrodermal activity) and adjustable ingame events (e.g., score system, difficulty, speed, graphics, sound) responding to the current physiological and psychological state of the exercising player. The proposed explorative design model for psychophysiological adaptable exergame fitness training for children is implemented in two interactive exergame concepts.

Keywords: Exergames, fitness training, psychophysiological adaption, dual flow, children

1   Introduction

Current physical activity and motion oriented games, based on entertainment consoles and multimedia interactions that require physical motion in order to play [1] are beginning to provide alternative ways to improve physical fitness. Additionally multimedia games can among others positively affect motivational, perceptual-motor and cognitive competencies [2].

Reviewing the existing research on game adjustments [e.g., 3] and on game-based motor learning [2], it seems to be highly promising to improve a child's physical fitness and cognitive growth by way of an exergame. Thus, the exergame design needs to be adaptive in a holistic and psychophysiological manner even when the exercising player gets used to the gameplay process. A sustainable exergame should provide a challenge accessible to players at different levels of fitness, age as well as gender and encourage the user continuously to a long-term program of activity.

Beside commercial exergames (e.g., Nintendo Wii, Microsoft Xbox), which have the potential to improve physical fitness, at least at low levels [e.g., 2], the presented model focuses on the novel trend of full-body exergame fitness for children (e.g., www.exergamefitness.com).

2 Background

The innovative approach of psychophysiological adaption is based on the traditional theory of flow [4]. To get in the "flow zone" [5] the challenge of the game and the abilities of the player need to be balanced. If the player's abilities are too strong and the game's requirements are too low, the player will be underchallenged, feel bored and therefore no longer be within the flow zone. The other way around, the player will be overstrained and feel frustrated, which results again in being out of the flow zone. Sinclair et al. [6] expanded the traditional, psychological based flow model to the physiological component while playing exergames, the "dual flow". Thereby, the player always needs to be within the corridor of an optimal combination of physical and psychological challenge and skill, e.g., between boredom and anxiety to stay motivated and successful in playing.

In terms of psychophysiological measurements such as heart rate (HR), electro-encephalogram (EEG) and electrodermal activity (EDA) in the field of game research, various approaches could be successfully applied to evaluate gameplay experiences in an objective, continuous, real-time, non-invasive, precise, and sensitive way [7]. The other way around, these methods can also be used as input device and therefore as basis of an adaptive holistic exergame design [e.g., 3].

3 Concept and Model

Based on this state of the art, further considerations were taken into account. By means of the equation for calculating the individual HR_{max}

$$HR_{max} = 220 - age\ [8],$$

the following training levels can be identified [9]: The health zone (50-60% of HR_{max}), the fat burning zone (60-70% of HR_{max}), the aerobic zone (70-80% of HR_{max}) and the anaerobic zone (80-90% of HR_{max}). Four thresholds are set in order to define the transition from one zone to another and ensure to remain the player in his/her optimal training zone. Therefore, the HR is measured by a chest band (Polar®, H7) and its related iPhone® App (Polar Beat), which are directly connected with the game engine (Unity4®) by a specific middleware and provide real-time data transfer for the whole playing duration. The same is established for a portable EEG sensor, which measures the player's emotional state. Therefore, three levels of emotional conditions are classified related to the flow concept: The "easy condition" is related to the psychological state of boredom, the "medium condition" to engagement and the "hard condition" to anxiety [e.g., 3].

In comparison with the target state, the player is guided to his/her optimal "dual flow" state by appropriate ingame events. The ingame events or single game mechanics (e.g., score system, difficulty, speed, graphics, sound) must be designed gradually in order to offer an adaptive gameplay. When measuring a high emotional level of stress the game provides more "relaxing" and positive events (e.g., colors or lower speed and less events) and reduces controlled stress-related components in order to establish an individual well-feeling system for the player ("flow zone"). If the exercising player is physically overstrained or underchallenged, the game will react with an adaption of the physical effort and intensity requirements (providing less or more requirements) in order to re-establish the player to his/her optimal performance mode.

In advance of the first training session, each player needs to be divided according to several categories by individual classifications of his/her current motor-skills and cognitive abilities (e.g., high-level motor-skills and low-level cognitive abilities). This pre-classification is investigated by using reliable and validated tests and questionnaires. Thus, the perfect conditions for a real-time adaptive exergame are fulfilled.

4   Implementation & Prototype Development

Currently, the proposed explorative design model is implemented in two user-tested interactive exergame concepts for physical and cognitive training, which are designed by Bachelor graduates of the Zurich University of the Arts (Fig. 1).

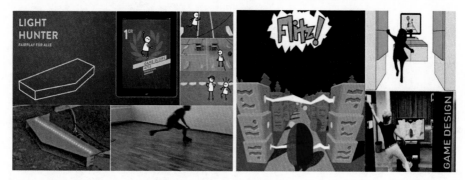

Fig. 1. Adaptive exergame prototypes "Light Hunter" and "Flitz!" (Source: ZHdK)

The single- and multiplayer exergame "Light Hunter" (by D. Mischler) consists of a "Light Hunter-App" for selecting the individual game mode and tracking one's scores. Moreover, it comprises single, portable, light-color-coded and interactive floor elements, which can be located in several spatial positions on the floor (in- and outdoor). By implemented distance-sensors, the elements react adaptive on the player's psychophysiological parameters resulting from moving and running through the game area predetermined by individual game tasks (e.g., frequency of tasks, color, sound). "Light Hunter" can be used in its standalone version as well as in addition with traditional training tools and exercises.

The single-player exergame "Flitz!" (by P. Pollinger & F. Osterwalder) consists of a motion-driven, height and width adjustable game controller and a virtual game scenario. The character moves through the virtual world in a third-person view. It has to overcome various obstacles, hit reward-items and avoid punishment-items by pushing the appropriate or mirrored (for cognitive training) of six specific positioned buttons surrounding the player's motion space. To control the game, the player has to move actively in three vertical (high, middle, low) and two horizontal directions (left and right). The game reacts adaptively to the player's psychophysiological parameters, by increasing or decreasing the difficulty of the game. The character speeds up, the range of motion gets wider as well as reward- and punishment-items appear more frequently in order to push the player's performance. The aim is to win as many points as possible within a specific time.

5   Outlook

Future work will focus on the evaluation of the prototypes in order to clarify the benefits of adaptive exergames in terms of physical and cognitive training for children. The impact of adaptive exergame fitness training on its effectiveness and attractiveness for the player will be investigated and compared with the outcomes of non-adaptive and traditional training within the framework of interdisciplinary study setups. This will result in the research-based modification of the prototypes and a generalizable player-centred design model for psychophysiological adaptive exergames, which might be used as a guideline for future game developments.

Acknowledgement. The authors want to thank D. Mischler, P. Pollinger and F. Osterwalder, R. Bauer and Prof. U. Götz from ZHdK as well as the Sportfond of the Canton Zurich (Swisslos) for their support.

References

[1] Oh, Y., Yang, S.: Defining Exergames & Exergaming, http://meaningfulplay.msu.edu/proceddings2010/mp2010_paper_63.pdf, (2010)

[2] Wiemeyer, J., Hardy, S.: Serious Games and motor learning - concepts, evidence, tech-nology. In: Bredl, K., Bösche, W. (eds.) Serious Games and Virtual Worlds in Education, Professional Development, and Healthcare, pp.197-220. IGI Global, Heshey, PA (2013)

[3] Chanel, G., Rebetez, C., Bétrancourt, M., Pun, T.: Emotion assessment from physiological signals for adaptation of game difficulty. In: IEEE Transactions on Systems, Man and Cybernetics, Part A: Systems and Humans, 41(6), pp. 1052-1063 (2011)

[4] Csikszentmihalyi, M.: Flow: The psychology of optimal experience. Harper Perennial, New York (1990)

[5] Chen, J.: Flow in games (and everything else). Communications of the ACM, 50(4), 31-34 (2007)

[6] Sinclair, J., Hingston, P., Masek, M.: Considerations for the design of exergames. In: Proceedings of the 5th International Conference on Computer Graphics and Interactive Techniques in Australia and Southeast Asia, pp. 289–295. ACM, New York (2007)

[7] Kivikangas, J. M., Ekman, I., Chanel, G., Järvelä, S., Cowley, B., Salminen, M., Henttonen, P., Ravaja, N.: Review on psychophysiological methods in game research. Proceedings of 1st Nordic DiGRA Digital Games Research Association (2010)

[8] Robergs, R.A., Landwehr, R.: The surprising history of the „HRmax=220-age" equation. Journal of Exercise Physiology online, 5 (2), 1-10 (2002)

[9] Gabriel, H., Wick, C., Puta, C.: Komponenten präventiven Gesundheitstrainings - Ausdauer, Kraft, Beweglichkeit, Koordination. In: Vogt, L., Neumann, A. (eds.) Sport in der Prävention: Handbuch für Übungsleiter, Sportlehrer, Physiotherapeuten und Trainer, pp. 33-65. Deutscher Ärzte-Verlag, Köln (2006)

A Serious Games platform for early diagnosis of mild cognitive impairments

Stefania Pazzi[1], Valentina Falleri[1], Stefano Puricelli[1], Daniela Tost Pardell[2], Ariel von Barnekow[2], Sergi Grau[2], Elena Cavallini[3], Sara Bottiroli[4], Chiara Zucchella[4] and Cristina Tassorelli[3,4]

[1]Consorzio di Bioingegneria e Informatica Medica – CBIM, Pavia, Italy
{s.pazzi, v.falleri, s.puricelli}@cbim.it
[2]Polytechnic University of Catalonia (UPC), Barcelona, Spain
ariel.von.barnekow@upc.edu - {dani,sgrau}@lsi.upc.edu
[3]Brain and Behavioral Sciences Department, University of Pavia, Italy
elena.cavallini@unipv.it
[4]C. Mondino National Neurological Institute, Pavia, Italy
sara.bottiroli@unipv.it - {chiara.zucchella,
cristina.tassorelli}@mondino.it

Abstract. Smart Aging, a Serious games (SGs) platform in a 3D virtual environment aimed at the early detection of Mild Cognitive Impairments (MCI) in persons ageing between 50 and 80. The navigation in a 3D environment (loft) that simulates in a reduced space the basic elements of interaction of home living, associated with the game approach results in a powerful screening tool, more friendly and motivating with respect to the traditional paper&pencil tests. The Smart Aging platform asks people to perform tasks related to daily activities, closer to real life than traditional paper&pencil tests, and, in doing so, it is able to evaluate different cognitive functions. The platform has been realized through a strong collaboration between game developers, neurologists and neuropsychologists. A scientific validation phase is ongoing on a sample of 1000 users to provide evidence of the efficacy and usefulness of the Smart Aging system.

Introduction

There is a general agreement on the idea that playing can boost brain functions and improve well-being [1,2]. Increasing evidence suggests that adults engaged in computer activities have decreased odds of developing MCI, defined as an intermediate stage between normal aging and dementia) [3]. Virtual reality-based memory training has provided promising results in preventing memory decline [4] and in reducing depression symptoms [5] in elderly adults. In particular, SGs potentially represent new and effective tools in the management and treatment of cognitive impairments in the elderly [6]. On the basis of this hypothesis and with the ambition of partially substituting pen-and-paper-based tests, we have designed and implemented Smart Aging, a web-based electronic test of MCI based on the SGs technology. Adoption of SGs in 3D virtual reality in the rehabilitative field favors the fast transfer of the acquired skills into real life, allows monitoring, control and documentation of the treatment effect, endless repetitions of the exercises and easiness of the implementation in a telematics scheme.

The virtual scenario

The Smart Aging platform provides a user-friendly treatment option to - *fill in electronic tests for the serial assessment of cognitive functioning (prevention, screening and early diagnosis). It also includes components for the self-training of cognitive functions at home with a 3D virtual environment presenting different scenarios for long-term preservation of cognitive function*

The 3D environment consists of a loft assembling in a reduced space the basic elements of interaction of a house: dining room, sitting room, bedroom and kitchen, plus a separate bathroom.

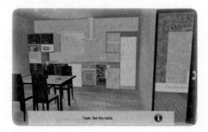

The game is based on a first-person paradigm so the player experiences the action through the eyes of an invisible avatar. The virtual position of the user within the environment is associated with a camera and the navigation model allows users to move within the environment at a constant height over the floor plane and to rotate the camera (head) within a limited range of angles.

Fig. 1 – The Smart Aging Virtual Scenario

The virtual environment is equipped with the following elements:
- *fixed elements that do not allow any interaction: walls, floor, ceiling, windows and decorative elements such as paintings, curtains and carpets;*
- *fixed elements that cannot be moved but can be used as a top to put and pick movable objects: bed, table, coach, kitchen marble, shelves;*
- *container elements with doors that can be opened and closed to put or get: kitchen cupboards, fridge and wardrobe;*
- *special interactive elements with specific functionalities: burners, sink;*
- *movable elements such as clothes, books and food.*

The platform tasks

The **Smart Aging SGs** require the performance of tasks related to daily activities, closer to real life than traditional paper&pencil tests (e.g. Mini Mental State Examination). The Smart Aging tasks have been designed in order to evaluate different cognitive functions: executive functions (reasoning and planning), attention (selected and divided), memory (short and long term, prospective), orientation (visuospatial). In the following Tab.1, the **Smart Aging Tasks** and the tested cognitive functions are summarized.

Task	Cognitive Functions
TASK 1 - OBJECTS IDENTIFICATION The subject is asked to identify and locate a list of objects in the kitchen.	Memory, spatial orientation and attention
TASK 2 – WATER THE FLOWERS WHILE LISTENING TO THE RADIO The subject is asked to turn on the radio and press the spacebar every time the word "sun" is aired, while watering the flowers on the windowsill.	Executive functions (planning), divided attention.
TASK 3 - MAKE A PHONE CALL TO ... The person is asked to make a phone call using the phone book and the phone placed on the night table next to the bed and then to turn the TV on.	Executive functions, selective attention, short/long-term and prospective memory.
TASK 4 - OBJECTS RECOGNITION A 2D screen with 24 images of objects is presented to the subject. The task is to identify the 12 objects that the subject was asked to identify in TASK 1.	Memory
TASK 5 - REPEAT THE OBJECTS IDENTIFICATION (TASK 1) The subject is is asked to find each of the objects that he looked for in TASK 1.	Long-term memory, spatial orientation, attention

Tab.1 – The Smart Aging Tasks

Before the beginning of the first task, the subjects perform a "familiarization" task. No other feedback is provided while the subjects are performing the games. An *Evaluation Index* is created based on the performance at the task, taking into account the number of correct actions, the number of errors, the omissions, the time needed to complete the task, the number of clicks and, finally, the distance travelled. The score of the SGs will be compared with traditional neuropsychological tests in order to validate the Smart Aging platform as a large scale screening tool for pre-symptomatic and early symptomatic assessment of cognitive impairments. The platform tasks are strongly customizable, in terms of number and type of objects to locate and time available for the different actions In the training component, the system features the possibility to select different levels of difficulty and a score counter, with the automatic upgrade to the next level when one reaches the threshold score. The playful characteristics of the platform are ensured by defining explicitly the goals of each task used to assess the performance of the player and by a positive/negative feed-back (right/wrong message at the end of the task).

The system navigation

The interface has been specially designed to make it accessible to older or non-expert users. Navigation in 3D is probably the more difficult type of manipulation for users without experience in 3D gaming. To make the task accessible for senior users, we have implemented an automatic navigation system. Users just need to click on the location where they want to go. The system computes automatically the best path to reach this location. The preliminary user tests showed that elderly users had difficulties in managing the mouse, therefore, we have implemented a touch-screen version of the interface. The selection is done by a touch gesture on the screen.

Indexes and validation

The game records all users actions. From these data, it computes a set of indices for each task of the game separately. At the end of the game these indices are parsed to give an overall score of the patient's cognitive skills. Currently, clinicians are working on the evaluation model, with the goal of making it equivalent to standardized measures based on paper and pencil screening tests. Recording all the indices provides flexibility in adjusting the model during the validation stage.

Conclusions

The system validation has already started: 1000 persons aged 50-80 are under evaluation for early detection of MCI. Subjects with confirmed MCI and/or neurodegenerative dementia will represent the secondary target group. Once validated, the Smart Aging SGs platform will constitute a powerful screening tool for the early detection of cognitive impairments on a wide scale. This approach has indeed several advantages as compared to the available screening tools for MCI: it is more friendly, ecological and motivating for the end-users, and it is less time- and resource-consuming for the professional figures.

References

[1] D. Bavelier, C. Green, D. Han, P. Renshaw, M. Merzenich, and D. Gentile. Brains on video games. Nature reviews Neuroscience, 12:763-768, 2012.

[2] S. Kuhn, T. Gleich, R. Lorenz, U. Lindenberger, and J. Gallinat. Playing super Mario induces structural brain plasticity: gray matter changes resulting from training with commercial video game. Molecular Psychiatry, 19:265-271, 2014.

[3] S. Negash, G. Smith, S. Pankratz, J. Aakre, Y. Geda, R. Roberts, D. Knopman, B. Boeve, R. Ivnik, and R. Petersen. Successful aging: Definitions and prediction of longevity and conversion to mild cognitive impairment. Am. J. Geriatr Psychiatry, 19(6):581-588, 2011.

[4] G. Optale, C. Urgesi, V. Busato, S. Marin, L. Piron, K. Priftis, L. Gamberini, S. Capodieci, and A. Bordin. Controlling memory impairment in elderly adults using virtual reality memory training: a randomized controlled pilot study. Neurorehabilitation and Neural Repair, 24(4):348-357, 2010.

[5] B. Fernandez Calvo, R. Rodriguez-Pérez, L. Contador, A. Rubio-Santorum, and F. Ramos. Efficacy of cognitive training programs based on new software technologies in patients with Alzheimer-type dementia. Psicothema, 23(1):348-357, 2010.

[6] E.P. Cherniack, Not just fun and games: applications of virtual reality in the identification and rehabilitation of cognitive disorders of the elderly. Disabil Rehabil Assist Technol, 6 (4) 283-289, 2011.

Requirements for an Architecture of a Generic Health Game Data Management System

Malypoeur Plong, Vero Vanden Abeele and Luc Geurts

e-Media Lab, Faculty of Engineering Technology, KU Leuven
A.Vesaliusstraat 13, 3000 Leuven, Belgium
{malypoeur.plong,vero.vandenabeele,luc.geurts}@kuleuven.be

Abstract. Often, logging data while playing a game-based health application is of specific interest, not only to the players themselves, but equally to therapists, health counselors, coaches, researchers, etc. Therefore, designing and developing a health game on its own is not enough; one also needs to foresee a health game *data management system* (DMS). In this paper we present eight requirements for a 'generic' health game DMS. We will start by discussing the diversity and similarity between four different health games and their data. After the analysis of the games and data, we will present a final set of requirements that need to be addressed when building a health game DMS: data-centralization, data-synchronization, data integrity, role-based access, accountability, a generic data structure, UI flexibility and development extensibility. We hope that these requirements can inform health game professionals when designing their own DMS.

Keywords. Games for health, data management system, health informatics

1 Introduction

The use of serious games in the field of health has witnessed a steep increase in the past years, as mentioned in [1, 2]. Ample attention has been given to games for health, and there are plenty of research studies that aspire to inform how to design health games [3, 4]. In addition, more and more of these games produce data that is of interest to the player and possibly to the coach, therapist or doctor. Data analytics of videogames has been a hot topic [5] and this is particularly pertinent to games for health as insight in player actions may provide insight in the assessment or rehabilitation process. However, when it comes to the *management of health game data* acquired during playing the game, not many related studies have been published. Obviously, there are plenty of studies on data management systems (DMS) in general, and the management of electronic health records in particular, as noted in [6]. However, the manner in which those general systems handle health records or manage data cannot readily be applied to game-based health applications because the type of data and the context differ.

Based on the analysis of four different health games and their idiosyncratic data management systems, this paper will discuss typical requirements when managing different kind of *health game data*. Secondly, from this analysis, requirements for a health game DMS will be introduced. Moreover, it is our aspiration that these requirements can result in a 'generic' health game DMS. Therefore, they can inform health game professionals how to design one DMS that can accommodate a variety of data logged from a variety of health games.

Games for health and their data

More and more, the logged data from players playing health application is of specific interest to clients, therapists, health counselors, coaches, researchers, etc. Hence, developing the game alone is not enough; one also needs to develop a data management system. Such a system should log and retrieve game data of every player, report and visualize the playing performance and perhaps even export the data in a preferable format. Only a few research studies describe how to build such a *health game* DMS. To the best of the author's knowledge, only one study was found [7] that focuses on player data management of health games, in particular upper limb rehabilitation with MS patients. And while building one dedicated game data management system is already daunting, it is even more challenging to build one system that can log and handle the data coming from a diversity of health games.

During the development of four different health games in our research lab (i.e. *Number Sense*, a game to train intuitive understanding of numbers in preschoolers, *DYSL-X* [8, 9], a game to aid in the assessment of dyslexia among preschoolers, *Visual Neglect* [10], a game to train psycho-motor skills and *stApp,* a game to mitigate sedentary behavior), it was noticed that each of these games relied on an idiosyncratic DMS notwithstanding that they were built for similar reasons and contained similar functionalities. Because of these idiosyncrasies, none of the system components were reusable for other projects. Differences were found in the type of logged data (time, duration, levels, scores, trials, etc.), individual player's information (name, location, institution, etc.), data visualization (graphs, tables, charts, etc.), data exportation format and especially the data access levels (who can see what data).

Obviously, designing and developing a different data management system for each health game increases costs and lengthens the development process. Moreover, with respect to maintainability, developing a separate DMS for each different health game might not be sustainable: data maintenance is never finished. As a consequence, the motivation to build one generic DMS for health data emerged. Such a generic DMS can synchronously log the data coming from multiple health games and accommodate data management of future games for health as well. In this paper we will present how we came up with the requirements for the health game DMS by discussing the diversity and similarity of health data that needed to be logged for four different games; where the games differed and where they presented similar needs. Next we will present a final set of requirements that need to be addressed when building a generic health game DMS. In a forthcoming paper, the actual architecture of such a health game DMS is discussed.

2   Games for health and their requirements

In the following paragraphs we discuss four different health games and the data management system that was required for each of these games.

2.1   DYSL-X

The aim of the DYSL-X project was to develop a game-based application to aid in the assessment of dyslexia among preschoolers. Therefore, the DYSL-X game encompasses three mini-games that embed psycho-acoustical tests, letter-recognition tasks (see Fig. 1) and end-phoneme recognition. These game-based assessments are administered at school, on an Android tablet with Wi-Fi connection. However, it was noticed during testing that stable internet connections at schools are not guaranteed.

User Roles. A school counselor most often administers the test; these tests are completed in approximately one hour. Right after completing the tests, the school counselor can make an assessment based on the results. Therefore, the data of the children should be accessible by the counselor. However, these counselors should only see the data of those children that they have tested themselves. In addition, researchers also want to have access to the data of these children for further research on dyslexia. In contrast to the school counselor, these researchers will not have access to the tablets at the different schools. Among researchers, we can distinguish further between research coordinators that want full access to all data of all children and job students that perhaps aid in collecting and/or analyzing data, but should only be able to 'read' the data, and certainly not edit or delete data. Furthermore, job students should only have access to data from certain groups of children. The research coordinator should be able to set these viewing rights of job students.

Types of Data. As aforementioned, the project consists of three mini-games: psycho-acoustical tests, letter-recognition tasks and end-phoneme recognition. Typical recorded data is amongst others the level and trial in the game, the difficulty setting, the choices offered to the player, the actual choice of the player and timestamps (see Table 1). Furthermore, demographic data of the player is recorded as well as specific information about the presence of dyslexia in the family.

Table 1. DYSL-X: health game data

Mini-games	Level	Trial	Playing data
Psycho-acoustical tests	1...n	1...n	Different frequencies of sound choices offered, correct choice, player's choice, difficulty level, display and response time
Letter-recognition	1...n	1...n	Different letters on display, correct choice, player's choice, display time and response time
End-phoneme recognition	1...n	1...n	Different items on display, reference item, correct item (ends with the same letter as reference item), player's choice, display time and response time

Table 2. DYSL-X: individual demographic player's data

	Player's information
Basic type	First name, last name, date of birth, tags (optional)
Survey type	Language, school, class, repeat grade, health problem, family problem, remarks

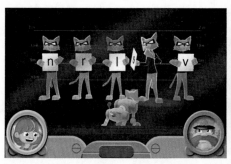
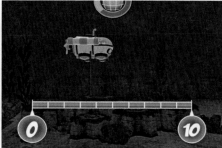

Fig. 1. DYSL-X project: mini-game that comprises the letter-recognition task.

Fig. 2. Number Sense project: mini-game that contains the number line task.

2.2 Number Sense

The Number Sense project aims to assess and remediate number sense in preschoolers. This is done via a suite of pretests and posttests (for assessment) and game applications (for training), designed for preschoolers and for children in grade three (age 8-9). The games run on Apple and Android tablets as well as PC. The suite contains 4 different mini-games involving *counting* numbers of dots, *connecting* numbers with groups of dots, *pointing at* a number on a number line (see Fig.2) and *comparing* different group sizes of dots. The games are administered at different locations such as care facilities, home or school. Similar to the DYSL-X project, internet connection at these locations cannot be guaranteed. In contrast with DYSL-X, the children play over an extended period of time. During several weeks, they play daily. In addition, they might play on a different platform than the day before.

User Roles. For this game, besides the individual player, the research coordinator is the only type of user. He or she should have full read/write access to all the information of every player, including basic demographic information, information from pretest and posttest and the data acquired during playing the mini-games. Furthermore, game data from different mini-games has to be exported in different formats (csv, excel, pdf).

Types of Data. Table 3 shows the game data from the Number Sense game. Its game data is organized in four different hierarchies: Session, Section, Level, and Trial. Table 4 illustrates the possible demographic data to be stored for the individual player.

Table 3. Number Sense on Android: health game data

Game Android	Session	Section	Level	Trial	Playing data
Counting dots	1...n	1...n	Pre,Post, Game	1...n	Stimulus value, player's answer, correct answer and reaction time
Connecting groups of dots to numbers	1...n	1...n	Pre,Post, Game	1...n	Stimulus value, number choices, player's answer, correct answer and reaction time
Pointing at Number Line	1...n	1...n	Pre,Post, Game Level {1...18}	1...n	Stimulus file, stimulus value, number choices, correct choice, player correctness in percentage, reaction time, PAE, scale, trial of experiment
Comparing different group sizes of dots	1...n	1...n	Pre, Post, Level, Game	1...n	Stimulus file left, stimulus file right, stimulus value left, stimulus value right, choices, correct choice, player's choice, ratio, distance, trial of experiment

Table 4. Number Sense: individual player data

	Player's information
Basic type	First name, last name, birthdate, birthplace, gender, school, year, field of study
Survey type	Mother's diploma, father's diploma and other bunch of survey questions

2.3   stApp

The stApp application is designed to inform users of the negative consequences of being seated for too long, and to make users stand up after half an hour of sitting (see Fig. 3)[11]. The application runs on an Android smartphone. It makes use of a separate motion sensor attached to the players' thigh, and the data acquired from sensor is communicated to a smartphone via Bluetooth. A mobile application then processes incoming data to define the user's state (sitting vs non-sitting). Users with good behavior will be rewarded by earning a high score and achievements. In addition, users can inspect their sitting versus standing behavior of the current and past days.

This application could be used at every possible place depending on where the user is: at home, work, or school, in the cinema, the restaurant or a sport center. It should be noticed that not every user has access to a mobile data network, and not every place provides Wi-Fi technology. Thus, a network connection is not always available. Again users will make use of stApp over an extended period of several weeks.

User Roles. The user will inspect his own progress via the application itself. In addition, the data acquired from the user's behavior is of interest to a research team that aims to study the effects between behavior and motivation. Therefore, the research team should have full read access to all the information of every user.

Types of Data. As depicted in Table 5, the data acquired from using the application is quite straightforward without a hierarchy. This is different from the previous health applications. In addition, Table 6 gives the basic demographic information of the individual user.

Table 5. stApp: logged game data

	Data from using application
Behavior during the day	Sitting time, sitting duration, standing time, standing duration, score achieved in each state, timestamp
Behavior end of the day	Achieved score of the day, achieved score of the day in percent
Achievements	Type of achievement rewarded

Table 6. stApp: individual demographic data

	User's information
Basic type	First name, last name, date of birth, profession, organization

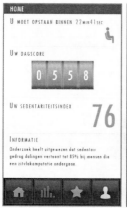

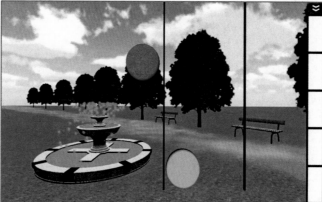

Fig. 3. stApp   **Fig. 4.** Visual Neglect: Screenshot of the Neglect Rehabilitation game

2.4   Visual Neglect

This game is developed for Android tablet, with the purpose of helping visual neglect patients (mostly elderly people) to rehabilitate (see Fig. 4)[10]. Patients are asked to follow and tap on a sphere that slowly moves further into their neglected field. In addition, more and more distracting visual elements are brought into the game as players progress through the different levels. This application can be used at the home of the patient or in care facilities. These patients will play the game daily over a period of several weeks.

User Roles. The patient with visual neglect (typically a senior that has suffered a stroke) has right to access to his/her own information: data from playing the game (Table 7) and basic demographic information (Table 8). Moreover, the therapist or clinician will also have full read/write access to all the information of his or her patient. Finally, the researchers from this project will equally have access to and be able to export those data with a preferable format, for statistical analysis as the underlying theory of multi-synchronicity (i.e. offering cross-modal stimuli that contain an auditory and visual channel and are in sync) is investigated through this game as well [12].

Types of Data. The application consists of an assessment to define the Center of Cancelation (CoC), which is a measure of the severeness of visual neglect. Based on the CoC the difficulty setting of the game is defined. In addition, there is the game itself that aims to train and mitigate visual neglect.

Table 7. Visual Neglect: health game data

Mini-game		Playing data
Neglect Assessment	Trial: 1…n	Image id, co-stimulus coordinates (x,y), co-stimulus type, number of clicked
	Level: 1…n	Image type, image size, rows, columns, score, level, lowest, highest
Neglect Rehabilitation	Trial: 1…n	Stimulus color change coordinates (x,y), tapping coordinates (x,y), ball coordinates on tap(x,y), reaction time
	Level: 1…n	Frequency, speed, number of balls, number of clicks, level, if level complete, play time, score

Table 8. Visual Neglect: individual player data

	Player's information
Basic type	First name, last name, date of birth, tags (optional)

3 Architecture requirements

When analyzing the aforementioned projects, the different data types and hierarchies become obvious, as well as the different user roles. Nevertheless, some generic requirements also come to the foreground. In order to have a system that is able to handle multiple game-based health applications, it is at least required to have the following eight main essential criteria: data-centralization, data-synchronization, data integrity, role-based access, accountability, generic data structure, UI flexibility and development extensibility. These eight requirements will be discussed in more detail.

Data-centralization

The assessment tests and games are played on a myriad of devices, even within one game. Therefore, all game data from different players should not only be stored locally but also be centralized on a central server. One or more clients—in this case game applications running on tablets or PCs can make a connection to this central server and exchange data when online. Furthermore, a central server can deliver data to a web-based *view of the data* so that therapists, doctors, researchers or coaches can view the game data as well, at any time and any place, without needing access to the actual tablet, smartphone or PC that was used to administer the test or play the game.

Data-synchronization

In many cases the game-based health application is played at locations where internet connection is limited. Hence, game data might not be sent to server in real time. Therefore, data logged during playing the game should first be stored locally on the user's device (smartphone, tablet, PC), and only be synchronized to the central server when an internet connection becomes available. Sufficient detail should be given to *when* synchronization is carried out, as synchronization slows down game-play. Having to wait until data is synchronized can ruin the game experience.

Data-integrity

Safeguarding the game data is paramount. Game data is sensitive and related to a person's health. Data that is lost or transformed during transmission could lead to wrong assumptions about one's health, and to errors in assessment and diagnosis. Moreover, data is also often used for scientific purposes. Therefore, during synchronization over the network from clients to the central server, measures need to be taken not to lose data. Procedures should be in place that can verify the integrity of the data and that can prevent data from being removed from the local device in case synchronization failed. At the same time, because of the need for safeguarding data, it is important to store data centrally, on a backed-up server, and not only locally, on a device that can crash.

Role-based access

Data of serious games is of interest to the individual player, as well as the coach/parent/therapist/researcher. However, data collected during playing games for health should be considered as confidential information, implying that all of player's information is *not* permitted to be viewed, let alone be edited, by everyone. Hence, different user-roles need to be established that need different access rights. These access rights include both limitations on viewing data as well as limitation on actions performed on the data. At least the following roles can be found in all systems:

Individual player: a player should have access to viewing his/her data from using the health application, but not be able to change his data.

Supervisor: a supervisor has read/write access to players' data, but only of that specific group of players that fall directly under his or her supervision.

Project researcher: a project researcher has read/write access to players' data, but only of that of specific group of players assigned by the project coordinator.

Project Coordinator: the top role of each health application. The project coordinator can create aforementioned users in lower hierarchy, grant them access rights and has full read/write access to all game data from all players belonging to that health application. Often this is a professor or researcher that is interested in the data for further research purposes.

General game data manager: in the case of one generic architecture, for multiple projects, a general game data manager is necessary: responsible for managing technical aspects of the systems (setting up a new health application, creating project coordinator, but has no access to the game data in any specific health application).

Accountability

Since these systems deal with confidential and health related data, monitoring every user roles' activities on the system is necessary for accountability. It should be recorded who views/edits which data. Because some activities performed by some user roles in the system can bring changes to the player's information, those activities should be intercepted and reported to the top user-role, i.e., project coordinator.

Generic data structure

Different health game applications store different types of data, e.g. response times, chosen items, stimulus coordinates, etc., and individual's demographic data, e.g. parent's diploma, family's problem, individual's health status, etc. While data diverges, within game based environments, generally, reaction times or durations matter. Hence timestamps that go along with user actions are pertinent. Therefore, a flexible design structure is necessary that suites the different types of data coming from multiple game-based health applications. In addition, most game-based data is contained within a hierarchy of sessions, levels, trials and finally difficulty settings. Hence, a generic system not only needs flexibility with respect to the different types of data, but equally with respect to different hierarchies of data. Moreover, such a system should be able to handle a large amount of game data efficiently: adding new data, updating existing data and retrieving data from the system should be performed at a high speed.

UI Flexibility

This term refers mainly to a flexible functionality in the system in adapting its view, based on the GUI configuration for disclosing the data, and for editing the data. From one game project to another, and from one user role to another, the differences can be the terminology, user actions, user roles and data formats. The system should be capable to adjust the view accordingly.

Development extensibility

Finally, new health game applications should easily be integrated to the system without making big changes to the core implementation. Building a separate health DMS for different game project should not be needed. Therefore, a modular structure should be devised with respect to the business logic as well.

4 Conclusion and Future works

While there is plenty of research in health informatics, and particularly within the domain of patient health records, there is a dearth of research that pertains to how to setup health game data management systems. This paper is a first attempt to address this void. Upon the analysis of four different health game applications, this paper introduced eight requirements for a generic system architecture that can handle multiple health games: data-centralization, data-synchronization, data integrity, role-based access, accountability, generic data structure, UI flexibility and development extensibility. Currently, we are continuing our investigations. In particular we have implemented such a generic health game DMS based on the above-mentioned requirements. However, given the scope of this paper, the discussion of the technical realization was not entailed in this paper but will be presented in a future article. We hope that these requirements can inform health game professionals how to design sustainable data management systems.

5   References

[1]   Ferguson, B.: The Emergence of Games for Health. Games Health J. 1, 1–2 (2012).

[2]   Gekker, A.: Health Games. In: Ma, M., Oliveira, M.F., Hauge, J.B., Duin, H., and Thoben, K.-D. (eds.) Serious Games Development and Applications. pp. 13–30. Springer Berlin Heidelberg (2012).

[3]   Deen, M., Schouten, B.A.: Games That Motivate To Learn: Design Serious Games By Identified Regulations. Improv. Learn. Motiv. Educ. Games Multidiscip. Approaches Hershey Idea Group Ref. (2011).

[4]   Sturm, J., Tieben, R., Deen, M., Bekker, T., Schouten, B.: PlayFit: Designing playful activity interventions for teenagers. Proceedings of DIGRA. pp. 14–17 (2011).

[5]   Seif El-Nasr, M., Drachen, A., Canossa, A.: Game Analytics - Maximizing the Value of Player Data. Springer Link (2013).

[6]   Chen, R.: Towards interoperable and knowledge-based electronic health records using archetype methodology. Linköping University Electronic Press, (2009).

[7]   Notelaers, S., De Weyer, T., Raymaekers, C., Coninx, K., Bastiaens, H., Lamers, I.: Data Management for Multimodal Rehabilitation Games. 2010 Workshop on Database and Expert Systems Applications (DEXA). pp. 137–141 (2010).

[8]   Audenaeren, L.V. den, Celis, V., Abeele, V.V., Geurts, L., Husson, J., Ghesquière, P., Wouters, J., Loyez, L., Goeleven, A.: DYSL-X: Design of a tablet game for early risk detection of dyslexia in preschoolers. In: Schouten, B., Fedtke, S., Bekker, T., Schijven, M., and Gekker, A. (eds.) Games for Health. pp. 257–266. Springer Fachmedien Wiesbaden (2013).

[9]   Celis, V., Husson, J., Abeele, V.V., Loyez, L., Van den Audenaeren, L., Ghesquière, P., Goeleven, A., Wouters, J., Geurts, L.: Translating preschoolers' game experiences into design guidelines via a laddering study. Proceedings of the 12th International Conference on Interaction Design and Children. pp. 147–156. ACM, New York, NY, USA (2013).

[10]   Stienaers, M., Tierens, M.: Automated assessment and game-based rehabilitation of visual neglect following brain injury, (2014).

[11]   Hamilton, M.T., Healy, G.N., Dunstan, D.W., Zderic, T.W., Owen, N.: Too little exercise and too much sitting: Inactivity physiology and the need for

new recommendations on sedentary behavior. Curr. Cardiovasc. Risk Rep. 2, 292–298 (2008).

[12]   Van Ee, R., van Boxtel, J.J., Parker, A.L., Alais, D.: Multisensory congruency as a mechanism for attentional control over perceptual selection. J. Neurosci. 29, 11641–11649 (2009).

Autonomous and Controlled Motivation in a Randomized Controlled Trial Comparing School-based and Computerized Depression Prevention Programs.

Marlou Poppelaars[1], Yuli R. Tak[1], Anna Lichtwarck-Aschoff[1], Rutger C.M.E. Engels[1,2], Adam Lobel[1], Sally N. Merry[3], Mathijs F. G. Lucassen[3], and Isabela Granic[1]

[1]Behavioural Science Institute, Radboud University Nijmegen, P.O. Box 9104, 6500 HE Nijmegen, The Netherlands.
{m.poppelaars, y.tak, a.lichtwarck-aschoff, r.engels,
a.lobel}@pwo.ru.nl
[2]Trimbos-Institute, P.O. Box 725, 3500 AS Utrecht, The Netherlands.
rengels@trimbos.nl
[3]Department of Psychological Medicine, Faculty of Medical and Health Sciences, University of Auckland , Private Bag 92019, Auckland 1142, New Zealand.
{s.merry, m.lucassen}@auckland.ac.nz

Abstract. The depression prevention video game SPARX was shown to be equally as effective as the classroom-based depression prevention program 'Op Volle Kracht' (OVK) in reducing depressive symptoms among adolescents girls. Because video games are known for their engaging qualities, this study examined possible motivational benefits of SPARX compared to OVK. No differences in autonomous and controlled motivation were found between conditions at any time point. However, OVK was negatively associated with autonomous motivation during the program, while SPARX and the OVK and SPARX combined were associated negatively with controlled motivation during the programs. Additionally, autonomous motivation and controlled motivation at the start of the interventions and controlled motivation half-way through the interventions was found to positively influence long-term depressive symptoms. Results indicate that depression prevention programs including video games can beneficially influence motivation. Further research is needed to delineate the effects of video game prevention programs on motivation.

Keywords: adolescents · depression prevention · video games

1 Introduction

Over the years, video games have become increasingly popular among adolescents, with almost all adolescents playing video games regularly [1,2]. Interestingly, video games have been shown to be capable of teaching adolescents a range of skills [e.g. 3] while simultaneously engaging youth in an activity they enjoy and seek out themselves. Moreover, it has been found that video games can increase positive mood and that players may regulate their mood through gameplay [4,5]. Thus, it is possible that not only cognitive skills but also emotional skills can be learned through video games [6].

One area of adolescent well-being that can potentially be addressed through video games is depression. Depression is one of the leading causes of disease burden [7] and even subclinical depressive symptoms cause significant impairment in school performance and social interactions [8]. Additionally, subclinical depressive symptoms are an important risk factor for major depressive disorder [9]. Prevalence of subclinical depression is estimated between 20% and 50% [10,11].

Most evidence-based depression prevention programs utilize Cognitive Behavioral Therapy (CBT) principles and are provided in didactic group settings [12]. Although these programs are effective on average [12,13], they suffer from a number of drawbacks, including high costs, potential stigmatization and limited accessibility for some youth who need it the most.

To address these limitations, more and more computerized prevention and intervention programs in the area of depression are being developed [14]. These programs aim to provide low cost interventions that are attractive to adolescents [15]. One promising example is the depression intervention video game SPARX [15,16]. SPARX was developed to decrease depressive symptoms in adolescents and may prevent depression by encouraging adolescents to actively practice CBT principals in an engaging format [15]. Thus, SPARX utilizes the same principles as many traditional depression prevention programs although its format is radically different.

Importantly, the first studies on SPARX have shown promising effects. Merry and colleagues [15] found SPARX to be equally as effective in reducing depressive symptoms as active treatment for adolescents with depressive symptoms. Additionally, Fleming, Dixon, Frampton and Merry [16] showed that SPARX decreased depressive symptoms compared to a waitlist-control condition in adolescents with probable depression. Finally, SPARX was shown to decrease depressive symptoms in adolescent girls with subclinical depressive symptoms equal to a traditional classroom-based program Op Volle Kracht (OVK) and an active monitoring control [17]. OVK is the Dutch adaptation of the most researched traditional depression prevention program, the Penn Resiliency Program, and has been found to be effective in a previous selective prevention study [18].

Besides studying whether video games such as SPARX can be effective in reducing depressive symptoms, it is important to research possible motivational benefits of depression prevention video games compared to traditional programs. As stated previously, video games are an immersive activity that the vast majority of adolescents engage in voluntarily; in other words, they are autonomously motivated to play. This is not surprising as video games are designed to attract players and encourage players to continue playing. Many basic game mechanics may be identified that are geared towards sustaining autonomous motivation during game play (e.g. points and levels). Although SPARX was mainly developed to teach CBT principles, the game was also developed, to improve engagement in therapy and stimulate players' autonomous motivation to play through in-game goals and rewards.

Self-determination theory posits that autonomous motivation, defined in this context as motivation stemming from interest or emotional satisfaction, apart from external rewards, is essential for treatment success [19]. Evidence shows that autonomous motivation leads to treatment gains and intention to persist in treatment [20]. For depression, more autonomous motivation has also been associated with better treatment outcomes and higher rates of remission [19, 20]. In contrast, controlled motivation (motivation stemming from pressure from others or internal pressure such as guilt) was found to negatively influence treatment outcomes and remission [19].

The current study investigated the differences in motivation between four interventions - SPARX, OVK, a combined OVK and SPARX program and a monitoring intervention - in adolescent girls with subclinical depressive symptoms. It was expected that autonomous motivation would increase and controlled motivation would decrease in participants playing SPARX (either with or without the OVK program). Alternatively, the support offered by the group setting of OVK may have also stimulated an increase of autonomous motivation and a decrease of controlled motivation, potentially showing the combination of the two programs was most beneficial for treatment motivation. In addition, it was expected that higher levels of autonomous motivation and lower levels of controlled motivation would predict lower levels of depressive symptoms one year after the interventions. Understanding motivational differences between depression prevention programs may help create more attractive and more effective depression prevention programs in the future.

2   Method

2.1   Sample and Procedure

Adolescent girls ($n = 962$) in the first two years of seven secondary schools in the Netherlands were screened, using the *Reynolds Adolescent Depression Scale* (RADS-2) [21]. Screening took place at the schools of participants during school hours. Parents gave passive consent for screening. The 30% of girls receiving the highest depression scores on the RADS-2 (RADS-2 score ≥ 59) were eligible for the study. Participants who indicated suicidal ideation (score 3 on Children's Depression Inventory item 9) or that they were receiving mental health care currently were excluded from the study. In total, 208 girls (*M*age = 12.83 years, $SD = 0.76$) participated with active consent from both the adolescents and their parents. Participants were randomly assigned to one of four conditions (SPARX $n = 51$, OVK $n = 50$, OVK & SPARX $n = 56$ and a monitoring condition $n = 51$) by an independent researcher. In order to obtain reasonable group sizes for the OVK and OVK & SPARX conditions, the amount of conditions was predetermined for each school and randomization was done separately for each school. Scores on depressive symptoms did not significantly differ between conditions at screening ($F(3, 204) = 2.08, p = .10$).

2.2   Interventions

Girls allocated to the SPARX condition played SPARX approximately once a week at their homes during the intervention period. SPARX is an interactive fantasy game that applies CBT principles to target depression. The game consists of seven levels in which CBT principles are introduced through interactive conversations with a guide and practiced with both in-game and real-life challenges. The OVK condition entailed a weekly classroom-based program provided by professional psychologists. In groups of ten to fifteen girls, participants received the first eight lessons of the OVK program. These lessons teach knowledge and skills to change maladaptive cognitions. The combined condition of OVK and SPARX consisted of 8 sessions of OVK and the scheduled SPARX play. The monitoring control condition only received weekly questionnaires during the intervention period. These weekly questionnaires, measuring depressive symptoms and daily stressors, were administered online to all participants.

2.3   Measures

The *Autonomous and Controlled Motivations for Treatment Questionnaire* (ACMTQ) [22] was adapted to the context of depression prevention program for adolescents. Participants rate twelve reasons which complete the sentence 'I participate in the resiliency training because …' on a seven-point scale (*strongly disagree* to *strongly agree*). Sample items are 'It is consistent with my life goals' (autonomous motivation) and 'I want others to approve of me' (controlled motivation). Cronbach's alpha was 0.87 for the subscale autonomous motivation at all three measurements (screening, pre-test and halfway through the programs) and ranged from 0.81 to 0.85 for the subscale controlled motivation.

Depressive symptoms were measured with the *Reynolds Adolescent Depression Scale* (RADS-2) [21] weekly during the intervention period and at 3, 6 and 12 months follow-up. The RADS-2 consists of 30 items (e.g. I feel sad) rated on a four-point scale (*almost never* to *most of the time*). Psychometric properties of the RADS-2 are reported to be good [21]. Girls received 50€ in total for their participation.

3   Results

At baseline (T0) all conditions were equal on education ($\chi^2(3, n = 208) = 0.71, p = .87$), age ($F(3, 204) = 1.34, p = .26$), ethnicity ($\chi^2(3, n = 208) = 0.19, p = .98$), religion ($\chi^2(3, n = 208) = 1.20, p = .75$), and gaming frequency ($F(3, 204) = 1.11, p = .35$). Therefore, baseline levels of these demographic variables were not included in the analyses as covariates.

ANOVA analyses showed that autonomous motivation did not differ between conditions at screening, pre-test and mid-test (Table 1). Similarly, controlled motivation did not differ between conditions at screening, pre-test and mid-test.

Table 1. Descriptives (Means and Standard Deviations) and F-values for ACMTQ Autonomous Motivation (AM) Controlled Motivation (CM) Scores per Condition at T0, T1 and T5.

	Control		OVK		SPARX		OVK & SPARX		F
	M	(SD)	M	(SD)	M	(SD)	M	(SD)	
AM T0	4.18	(1.18)	3.99	(1.30)	4.19	(1.51)	4.18	(1.35)	0.27
AM T1	4.59	(0.93)	4.80	(1.27)	4.29	(1.50)	4.47	(1.20)	1.44
AM T5	4.38	(0.94)	3.92	(1.46)	4.30	(1.45)	4.24	(1.39)	1.08
CM T0	2.62	(1.31)	2.56	(1.12)	2.34	(0.99)	2.82	(1.32)	1.42
CM T1	2.21	(0.94)	2.24	(0.97)	2.41	(1.14)	2.49	(1.35)	0.72
CM T5	2.36	(1.06)	2.22	(1.31)	2.00	(1.08)	2.17	(1.41)	0.74

Next, to test if conditions differed in their changes in motivation over time Repeated Measures ANOVAs were performed for autonomous and controlled motivation separately. Figure 1 and 2 show the trajectories from pre-test to mid-test of autonomous motivation and controlled motivation respectively. For autonomous motivation the Huynh-Feldt correction was used, because the assumption of sphericity was violated according to the Mauchly's test $\chi2$ (2) = 16.85, $p < 0.001$, $\varepsilon = .95$. A significant main effect of time on autonomous motivation was found between T0 and T5 ($F(1.89, 1.00) = 9.99$, $p < .001$). Within-Subjects contrasts indicated a quadratic effect ($F(1, 193) = 25.58$, $p < .001$). As can be seen in Figure 1, autonomous motivation increases before the start of the interventions and decreases during the interventions. Furthermore, there was a significant interaction between time and condition ($F(5.67, 3.00) = 2.48$, $p < .01$), showing that conditions differed in their change over time. As can be seen from Figure 1, OVK shows a sharper increase in autonomous motivation before the start of the treatments, followed by a sharper decrease during treatment compared to the other conditions.

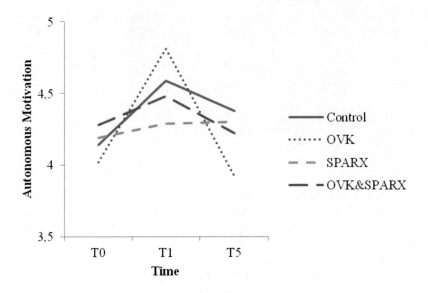

Fig. 1. Trajectories of mean autonomous motivation scores by condition.

For controlled motivation the Huynh-Feldt correction was used again (Mauchly's test $\chi2$ (2) = 21.26, $p < 0.001$, $\varepsilon = .93$). A significant main effect of time on controlled motivation was found between T0 and T5 ($F(1.86, 1.00) = 12.02$, $p < .001$). Within-Subjects contrasts indicated a linear effect ($F(1, 193) = 20.65$, $p < .001$), indicating an overall decrease in controlled motivation over time (see Figure 2). Additionally, there was a interaction between time and condition on a trend level ($F(5.56, 3.00) = 1.89$, $p = .09$), suggesting that conditions showed different changes over time. Figure 2 suggests that the overall decrease in controlled motivation is larger for the OVK & SPARX condition than the other conditions.

Besides testing whether there were group differences in motivation over time, we tested if the interventions influenced a change in motivation specifically during the programs. Therefore, regression analyses were performed predicting motivation at mid-test while controlling for motivation at pre-test. OVK was negatively associated with autonomous motivation half way through the program when controlling for pre-test levels of autonomous motivation ($b = -0.60$, $t(192) = -2.81$, $p < .01$). Both the SPARX ($b = 0.12$, $t(192) = 0.57$, $p = .57$) and the OVK & SPARX ($b = -0.08$, $t(192) = -0.40$, $p = .69$) conditions did not influence autonomous motivation at mid-test. Thus, participants in the OVK condition showed a relative decrease in their autonomous motivation, while participants in the SPARX and OVK & SPARX condition remained stable in their autonomous motivation.

Furthermore, controlled motivation half-way through the interventions was negatively associated with both SPARX ($b = -0.50$, $t(192) = -2.64$, $p < .01$) and OVK & SPARX ($b = -0.45$, $t(192) = -2.38$, $p < .05$) when controlling for pre-test. While OVK

(b = -0.16, $t(192)$ = -0.82, p = .41) had no effect on controlled motivation at mid-test when controlling for initial controlled motivation. Participants in the SPARX and OVK & SPARX conditions therefore showed a relative decrease in their controlled motivation, while the participants in the OVK condition remained stable in their controlled motivation.

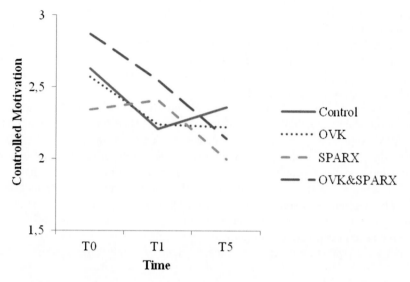

Fig. 2. Trajectories of mean autonomous motivation scores by condition

Furthermore, we tested whether autonomous and controlled motivation were associated with long-term depressive symptoms one year after the interventions. Autonomous motivation at the start of the interventions (T1; b = 1.42, $t(189)$ = 1.76, p = .08) was associated positively with depressive symptoms at one year follow-up at a trend level when controlling for baseline symptoms. However, autonomous motivation half-way through the interventions (T5; b = 0.58, $t(198)$ = 0.76, p = .45) was not associated with depressive symptoms at one year follow-up. Thus, participants who reported more autonomous motivation at the start of the program reported more depressive symptoms one year later, although this effect did not hold up for autonomous motivation at mid-test. Controlled motivation at pre-test was associated with depressive symptoms at one year follow-up at a trend level when controlling for depressive symptoms at screening (b = 1.77, $t(189)$ = 1.55, p = .07). In addition, controlled motivation half-way through the interventions, controlled for baseline depressive symptoms, was associated negatively with depressive symptoms at one year follow up (b = 1.96, $t(189)$ = 2.30, p < .05). Thus, participants who reported less controlled motivation at the start and half-way through the interventions seemed to have less depressive symptoms one year after the interventions independent of their baseline depressive symptoms.

4   Discussion

Absolute values of autonomous and controlled motivation did not differ between the conditions at any time point. Additionally, differences in group means over time were assessed for the conditions. It was shown that autonomous motivation increased before the start of the programs and decreased during the programs. This effect was strongest for the OVK condition, possibly indicating that expectations of the classroom-based program were particularly positive. Furthermore, controlled motivation was shown to decrease from screening to mid-test, indicating that internal and external pressure to participate was experienced less. This effect appeared strongest for the combined OVK and SPARX condition.

Moreover, influences of the interventions on changes in controlled and autonomous motivation were studied. Results indicated that SPARX and the combined OVK and SPARX program were not associated with changes in autonomous motivation during the programs, while these conditions did have a negative effect on controlled motivation half-way through the program. In contrast, the OVK condition had a negative influence on autonomous motivation during the programs and no effect on controlled motivation. Autonomous and controlled motivation at the start of the interventions and controlled motivation half-way through the interventions positively predicted long-term depressive symptoms one year after the interventions. These results need to be interpreted with caution, because changes in motivation scores were very small.

The current results support the idea that SPARX helps decrease controlled motivation. One explanation for this effect could be that participants were free to choose when they played SPARX. Additionally, within the program participants were given some freedom to choose their own path and their own way to play the game (e.g. create their own avatar and experiment with response options in conversations with game characters). This may have decreased feelings of outside pressure to participate in the program. Furthermore, although SPARX did not increase autonomous motivation during the program, SPARX may have prevented a decrease in autonomous motivation as was seen in the OVK condition. On the other hand, levels of autonomous motivation in the conditions with SPARX were not very high, suggesting that there was definite room for improvement. Possibly the didactic content of the game, stemming from its aim to teach CBT principles, overshadowed the attractive elements of game play. Although SPARX contains basic game mechanisms to create an engaging game play experience, more emphasis on mechanics that foster agency and a sense of exploration an discovery during game play may be needed to allow for increases in autonomous motivation. Further research is needed to examine which elements of SPARX influence motivation and how these elements may be improved to stimulate autonomous motivation.

In addition, it is unclear at this point how motivation developed after the first half of the interventions. For example, the negative influence of OVK on autonomous motivation during the program may have been a temporary dip in motivation. Treatment of psychopathology is hard and symptom improvement is not always linear [24, 25, 26]. Possibly the trajectory of motivation for treatment is also non-linear and a dip is to be expected for autonomous motivation mid-treatment, as participants may feel challenged in their belief that the intervention will help them. Future research is encouraged to include motivation measures closer to the end of interventions.

Although no absolute differences in mean motivation were found in any of the conditions, it was shown that lower levels of controlled motivation at the start and half-way through the interventions predicted less depressive symptoms one year after the interventions. Thus, ensuring low levels of controlled motivation may be essential for treatment outcomes. The influence of controlled motivation on depressive symptoms has also been found by Zuroff and colleagues [19]. However, our current study results were not consistent with earlier results on the beneficial influence of autonomous motivation on treatment results [19, 20]. Possibly, the positive association of autonomous motivation at the start of the interventions with long-term depressive symptoms is a result of the need for the program.

The present study was the first to study the motivational benefits of a video game based depression prevention program compared to a classroom-based depression prevention program. Results indicate that depression prevention programs including video game play can beneficially influence motivation. This is promising as lower controlled motivation was shown to be predictive of long-term lower depressive symptoms and earlier research has shown that autonomous motivation during treatment predicts better treatment outcomes and persistence in treatment. Further research is needed to determine which game elements are beneficial for motivation and how video game based interventions may be adjusted to optimize motivation.

References

[1] Dorsselaer S. van, Zeijl E., Eeckhout S. van den, Bogt T. ter, Vollebergh, W.: HBSC 2005: Gezondheid en Welzijn van Jongeren in Nederland. Trimbos-instituut, Utrecht (2007)

[2] Lenhart, A., Kahne, J., Middaugh, E., Macgill, A. R., Evans, C., Vitak, J.: Teens, Video Games, and Civics. Pew Internet & American Life Project, http://www.pewinternet.org/Reports/2008/Teens-Video-Games-and-Civics. aspx (2008)

[3] Green, C. S., Bavelier, D: Learning, Attentional Control, and Action Video Games. Current Biology 22, 197-206 (2012)

[4] Olson, C. K.: Children's Motivations for Video Game Play in the Context of Normal Development. Review of General Psychology 14 (2), 180-187 (2010)

[5] Ryan, R. M., Rigby, C. S., Przybylski, A: The Motivational Pull of Video Games: A Self Determination Theory Approach. Motivation and Emotion 30, 347-363 (2006)

[6] Granic, I., Lobel, A., Engels, R. C. M. E: The Benefits of Playing Video Games. American Psychologist 69 (1), 66-78 (2013)

[7] Murray, C. J. L., Lopez, A. D.: Global Mortality, Disability, and the Contribution of Risk Factors: Global Burden of Disease Study. Lancet 349, 1436-1442 (1997)

[8] Gotlib, I. H., Lewinsohn, P. M., Seeley, J. R.: Symptoms Versus a Diagnosis of Depression: Differences in Psychosocial Functioning. Journal of Consulting and Clinical Psychology 63 (1), 90-100 (1995)

[9] Nolen-Hoeksema, S., Girgus, J. S.: The Emergence of Gender Differences in Depression During Adolescence. Psychological Bulletin 115 (3), 424–443 (1994)

[10] Kessler, R. C., Avenevoli, S., Merikangas, K. R.: Mood Disorders in Children and Adolescents: An Epidemiologic Perspective. Biological Psychiatry 49, 1002–1014 (2001)

[11] Petersen, A. C., Compas, B. E., Brooks-Gunn, J., Stemmler, M., Ey, S., Grant, K. E.: Depression in Adolescence. American Psychologist 48 (2), 155-168 (1993)

[12] Merry, S. N., Hetrick, S. E., Cox, G. R., Brudevold-Iversen, T., Bir, J. J., McDowell, H.: Psychological and Educational Interventions for Preventing Depression in Children and Adolescents (Review). Cochrane Database of Systematic Reviews 12, CD003380 (2011)

[13] Horowitz, J. L., Garber, J.: The Prevention of Depressive Symptoms in Children and Adolescents: A Meta-Analytic Review. Journal of Consulting and Clinical Psychology 74 (3), 401–415 (2006)

[14] Calear, A. L., Christensen, H.: Review of Internet-Based Prevention and Treatment Programs for Anxiety and Depression in Children and Adolescents. Medical Journal of Australia 192 (11), S12-S14 (2010)

[15] Merry, S. N., Stasiak, K., Shepherd, M., Frampton, C., Fleming, T., Lucassen, M. F. G.: The Effectiveness of SPARX, a Computerised Self Help Intervention for Adolescents Seeking Help for Depression: Randomised Controlled Non-Inferiority Trial. BMJ 344, e2598 (2012)

[16] Fleming, T., Dixon, R., Frampton, C., Merry S. N.: A Pragmatic Randomised Controlled Trial of Computerized CBT (SPARX) for Depression among Adolescents Alienated from Mainstream Education. Behavioural and Cognitive Psychotherapy 40 (5), 529-41 (2012)

[17] Poppelaars, M., Tak, Y. R., Lichtwarck-Aschoff, A., Engels, R. C. M. E., Lobel, A., Merry, S. N., Lucassen, M. F. G., Ganic, I.: A Randomized Controlled Trial Comparing a School-Based (Op Volle Kracht) and a Computerized (SPARX) Depression Prevention Program for Adolescent Girls with Subclinical Depression. Unpublished manuscript (2014)

[18] Wijnhoven, L. A. M. W., Creemers, D. H. M., Vermulst, A. A., Engels, R. C. M. E., Scholte, R. H. J.: Randomized Controlled Trial Testing the Effectiveness of a Depression Prevention Program ('Op Volle Kracht') among Adolescent Girls with Elevated Depressive Symptoms. Journal of Abnormal Child Psychology 42, 217-228 (2014)

[19] Zuroff, D. C., Koestner, R., Moskowitz, D. S., McBride, C., Marshall, M., Bagby, M.: Autonomous Motivation for Therapy: A New Common Factor in Brief Treatments for Depression. Psychotherapy Research 17 (2), 137-147 (2007)

[20] McBride, C., Zuroff, D. C., Ravitz, P., Koestner, R., Moskowitz, D. S., Quilty, L., Bagby, R. M.: Autonomous and Controlled Motivation and Interpersonal Therapy for Depression: Moderating Role of Recurrent Depression. British Journal of Clinical Psychology 49, 529–545 (2010)

[21] Reynolds, W.M.: Reynolds Adolescent Depression Scale: Professional Manual (2nd ed.). Psychological Assessment Resources, Inc., Odessa (2002)

[22] Zuroff, D. C., Koestner, R., Moskowitz, D. S., McBride, C., Ravitz, P.: [Responses to the ACMTQ of Depressed Outpatients Seen in an Interpersonal Therapy Clinic]. Unpublished raw data (2005)

[23] Graham, J. W.: Missing Data Analysis: Making it Work in the Real World. Annual Review of Psychology 60 (1), 549-576 (2009)

[24] Hayes, A. M., Feldman, G. C., Beevers, C. G., Laurenceau, J-P., Cardaciotto, L. A., Lewis-Smith, J.: Discontinuities and Cognitive Changes in an Exposure-based Cognitive Therapy for Depression. Journal of Consulting and Clinical Psychology 75 (3), 409–421 (2007)

[25] Hayes, A. M., Laurenceau, J-P., Feldman, G., Strauss, J. L., Cardaciotto, L. A.: Change is not Always Linear: The Study of Nonlinear and Discontinuous Patterns of Change in Psychotherapy. Clinical Psychology Review 27, 715-724 (2007)

[26] Tang, T. Z., DeRubeis, R. J.: Sudden Gains and Critical Sessions in Cognitive-Behavioral Therapy for Depression. Journal of Consulting and Clinical Psychology 67 (6), 894-904 (1999)

Meaningful Feedback at Opportune Moments: How persuasive feedback motivates teenagers to move

Janienke Sturm, Sander Margry, Muriel van Doorn, Wouter Sluis-Thiescheffer

Fontys University of Applied Science, Eindhoven, The Netherlands
j.sturm@fontys.nl, wouter.sluis@fontys.nl

Abstract. Teenagers spend a large proportion of their day doing sedentary activities. They sit in school during classes and breaks, and after school they sit while doing homework, watching television or playing computer games. Novel ways of stimulating teenagers to be more active include applying games and play, because of its intrinsically motivating value. This paper presents a qualitative study of the role of persuasive feedback in a physical activity game. We performed interviews with teenagers who used a running game for several weeks. We describe their attitude towards persuasive feedback, its perceived effectiveness and possibilities for improvement.

1   Introduction

Teenagers spend a large proportion of their day sedentary: In school they sit during classes, breaks and after school are often spend sitting while doing homework, watching television or playing computer games. Minimal levels of physical activity can have serious health consequences. To prevent that, many initiatives have been developed aiming to reduce sedentary behaviour and stimulating physical activity (Foster et al., 2013; NASB, 2012). Increasingly, these interventions apply elements of gaming and play, because children and teenagers are intrigued by computer games on consoles and smartphones. The fact that games are intrinsically motivating and that games have been designed to capture the attention of their players for a prolonged period of time, makes games ideal instruments for behaviour change interventions.

Persuasive feedback is one of the mechanisms often applied in games and other applications intended to change behaviour; it provides the player with feedback that is aimed at increasing or sustaining desired behaviour. This paper describes a qualitative study of the role of persuasive feedback in a physical activity game. We start out by introducing some basics of motivation, behaviour change and persuasive mechanisms. Subsequently, we describe the setup of the study and report the main insights regarding teenagers' attitude towards persuasive feedback in the game and its perceived effect. We conclude with some general implications for the design of persuasive feedback in physical activity games.

2   Theoretical background

2.1   Motivation

One of the most used motivation theories, the Self-Determination Theory (SDT, Deci & Ryan, 2000) focuses on the extent to which people's behaviour is self-motivated. It describes the factors that contribute to people making their own choices. SDT distinguishes intrinsic motivation – performing an activity because of interest or enjoyment in the task itself - and extrinsic motivation – performing an activity in order to attain a certain outcome. There are various forms of extrinsic motivation, varying in the degree to which a person has internalised the external influences. To achieve behaviour change, intrinsic motivation or the more internalised forms of extrinsic motivation are most effective. When people are intrinsically motivated they are more inclined to act and their effort will be larger than when their motivation is purely extrinsic. Extrinsic motivation creates only short-term behaviour change: when the external motivator is removed, the new behaviour is likely to disappear as well.

According to SDT, three basic ingredients contribute to the experience of intrinsic motivation: autonomy, competence and relatedness. Autonomy refers to the need to make one's own choices (for instance being able to choose between various types of exercises); relatedness is the need to interact with, be connected to and care for others (for instance having fun with fellow members of a fitness class); and competence is the need to feel able to and confident in performing a task (for instance experiencing success in a challenging physical exercise).

2.2   Persuasion and behaviour change

In his Behaviour Model, Fogg (2009) describes three elements that have to be sufficiently present for desired behaviour to occur: motivation, ability and triggers (or opportunity). Motivation has been described in section 2.1. Ability denotes whether a person is capable of performing certain behaviour and is strongly related to simplicity: how easy is it to perform the desired behaviour? Ability is determined by elements like time, physical effort, cognitive effort, etc. Triggers, finally, are a call to action towards people. Triggers are crucial elements in persuasion. Three types of triggers can be distinguished: *Sparks* (motivational messages); *Facilitators* (making it easier to perform the behaviour); and *Signals* (reminders).

Persuasive feedback is a trigger in either of these forms. It provides the user with information that can be used to decide whether or not to sustain the current behaviour, or to change direction. The timing of persuasive feedback is crucial: the right information should be provided at the most opportune moment. According to Fogg's behaviour model, providing feedback is most effective when it is done when a person is both motivated and able to perform the behaviour. The best timing of feedback is dependent on the type of feedback: for instance, performance feedback should be given immediately after the action has taken place.

3   Study setup

This study aimed to explore teenagers´ attitude towards persuasive feedback and its perceived effect in a physical activity game: *Zombies, Run!*. Zombies Run! is a commercially available running game to be played on a smartphone. Players have to complete a number of missions, during which they run while listening to various audio narrations that uncover the story. A GPS-tracker tracks their running pace, while moaning zombies force the players to increase their tempo to escape them. While running, players collect items that are used to equip the players' virtual base camp, adding an extra layer of interest beyond the burn rate of calories (Moses, 2012).

Several types of persuasive feedback can be identified in this game. *Sparks* are provided in the form of motivating messages such as "Good job, you did great!" and as performance feedback such as "You have to run faster; the zombies are gaining on you!". *Facilitators* appear in the form of help messages showing how to play the game. *Signals* are provided in the form of beeps that urge the player to run and the sound of the zombies. Another type of Signal was added manually by the researcher in the form of regular WhatsApp messages reminding the players to play the game.

We recruited nine students (aged 13 or 14) from two vocational schools in the Netherlands. All players took part voluntarily. They were asked to play the game individually during two weeks. After these two weeks, each of the students was interviewed in a semi-structured interview addressing their attitude towards the persuasive feedback in the game, the perceived effect of the feedback and possibilities for improvement of the game. All interviews were transcribed and then underwent open and axial coding.

4   Results and discussion

General: The students were free to choose the number of times they played. All students indicated they liked the game and they thought it improved their physical condition. The audio narrations were perceived to be fun and captivating. The zombies that chase the players in order to make them run, were considered both fun and realistic.

Attitude towards persuasive feedback: Sparks, in the form of positive feedback (for instance compliments about their achievements), were liked by eight students and stimulated them to play on. However, some students indicated that they would prefer this type of feedback to be more explicitly related to their performance. The amount of motivational (performance-related) feedback in the game was perceived to be limited. More motivational feedback would possibly lead to more long-term play. Facilitators, in the form of help messages at the start of the game, were not perceived to be useful. The students indicated that they would prefer these facilitators to be better integrated in the game, much like the general approach in current mobile games, in which the workings of the game are gradually explained while playing the first few levels of the game. Signals, in the form of WhatsApp reminders that were sent daily by the researcher, were appreciated by eight students; they reported that these messages stimulated them to play the game without feeling obliged to do so. However, several students indicated that too many push messages would be annoying.

Perceived effectiveness: Seven students indicated that the compliments encouraged them to continue running. Also, seven students reported that the panting sounds of the zombies made them increase their pace. Although the WhatsApp messages were appreciated, only two players indicated that they would start to play the game after receiving such a signal. It was noted by some students that the timing of these push messages is crucial, too many messages would be rather annoying than helpful. Eight students indicated that the game helped them to be more physically active during the evaluation period. In the interviews all students said that they would like to continue playing the game. After a month at least five students were indeed still playing.

Possible improvements: Several students found it important to have the option to set their own performance goals in the game (autonomy), and to receive performance feedback about the extent to which they achieved their goals (competence). All students indicated that an option to play together with other people would be highly motivating (relatedness). Finally, they would also like to be informed about the performance of their friends.

5   Conclusion

The qualitative study described explored teenagers' attitude towards a game aimed at stimulating people to be physically active and measured the perceived effect of persuasive feedback. The sample size of this study was rather small (n=9) and the findings may be specific to the game used. Nonetheless, the study resulted in interesting insights in what persuasive feedback students liked or not and to what extent persuasive feedback was effective. In this case study, it was very important that (1) motivational feedback provided is directly related to a player's performance and (2) that players can play with others and share their results.

References

[1] Deci, E. & Ryan, R. (2000) Self-determination theory and the facilitation of intrinsic motivation, social development, and well-being. American Psychologist, 55, 68-78.

[2] Fogg, B.J. (2009) "A behaviour model for persuasive design". Proceedings of Persuasive'09. April 26-29, Claremont, California, USA.

[3] Foster, C., Richards, J., Thorogood, M., Hillsdon, M. (2013) Remote and web 2.0 interventions for promoting physical activity. Cochrane Database of Systematic Reviews 2013, Issue 9.

[4] Moses, T. (2012) Zombies, Run! - review. The Guardian. Retrieved May 15, 2014 from http://www.theguardian.com/technology/2012/mar/25/zombies-run-naomi-alderman-app.

[5] NASB (2012) Interventieoverzicht 2011/2012. Internal Report Nationaal Actieplan Sport en Bewegen. Retrieved May 15, 2014, retrieved from http://www.nasb.nl/beweegprojecten/interventieoverzicht-2011-2012.pdf

Active Parks: 'Phygital' urban games for sedentary and older people

Emmanuel Tsekleves[1], Adrian Gradinar[1], Andy Darby[2], Marcia Smith[2]

[1]Imagination Lab, Design, Lancaster University, LA1 4YW, UK
e.tsekleves@lancaster.ac.uk, a.gradinar@lancaster.ac.uk
[2]Highwire Centre for Doctoral Training, Lancaster University, LA1 4YW, UK
a.darby@lancaster.ac.uk, m.smith10@lancaster.ac.uk

Abstract. We present our work in the Active Parks project, aimed at encouraging older and sedentary people to take casual physical exercise in urban spaces, such as parks. This is achieved through the co-design of playful 'phygital' (physical and digital) artefacts and games to be installed in the park. The initial testing of our proof-of-concept prototype received extremely positive feedback as a potential way of motivating people to keep active in the park and in bridging the generation gap.

Keywords: Playful design, Physical-digital interaction, Co-design, Urban games

1 Introduction

Green spaces, such as parks are seen as a key contributor to wellbeing and the environment and have a proven track record in reducing the impact of deprivation and delivering better health and wellbeing, adding to the creation of a stronger sense of community [1]. Several parks in the UK are currently underutilised, especially by sedentary and older people. In the Active Parks project we are exploring how to engage older and sedentary park users in taking casual physical activity through playful 'phygital' (physical and digital) interactions. Working together with local community groups who look after the park, the Lancaster City Council and NHS Lancashire Public Health, we have co-designed a playful 'digital health trail', which offers a new way of motivating and taking casual physical activity specific to local people in their park (using Ryelands Park in the city of Lancaster, in the UK as a use case).

2 Related Work

Playful design, the mapping of playful experiences from video games to other non-game context experiences, has gained interest in recent years with a number of models been investigated [2]. A number of 'phygital' urban games have been developed, which offer playful experiences. These focus on encouraging exploitation and discovery of urban spaces in a leisurely and playful manner by connecting the digital (mobile phones with GPS/NFC technologies) with the physical world (e.g. building, city landmarks) reporting positive results in increasing people engagement with such experiences [3–5]. Playful design has not been explored as widely though in engaging older and sedentary people with physical activity. The work of Romero et al. [6] is the closest to date as it employs playful experiences targeting older people in care home facilities by following a traditional user-centred design methodology. There is a great potential, therefore, to go beyond user-centred design and explore how more participatory design methodologies, such as co-design can create playful 'phygital' experiences that encourage sedentary and older people in taking casual physical activity [7] in public urban spaces, such as in parks.

3   The Co-design Process

Co-designing with users has the potential to be transformative as participants become co-owners of innovation, having a much higher stake in its design, making and ultimately use. A co-design process [8] incorporating a number of workshops and events in the park was the starting point of our research. In the co-design workshops the research team engaged with a small representative group of the community residents. The events in the park were aimed at capturing data from a wider range of people in the area and larger numbers of local residents to validating the outcomes of the co-design workshops.

The co-design activities were focused on capturing people's values, needs and aspirations on the type of physical activities they enjoy doing and would like to do in the park. In a subsequent workshop this led to a shared vision, namely: 'A community space with fun and activities safe for everyone to enjoy'. The key values identified by workshop participants were activities that are playful, that help bridge the generation gap, and ones that are accessible to everyone. Looking at the affordances (physical and digital technology resources) and constraints (e.g. park geography, weather) of creating an interactive and playful casual activity trail, our co-designers started generating rich ideas for potential activities. The best ideas were then taken forward in a creative session where workshop participants created prototypes (using low-fidelity prototyping tools) of the selected activities. These included a large 'phygital' xylophone style activity, where one exercises by moving around it to create music; a mobile phone generated zombie chase activity incorporating physical challenges in the park; a park discovery and exercise activity, where set challenges invite you to physically explore the park through interactive, enjoyable and playful stories.

4   Making of the Proof-of-concept Prototype

From these the one, which the research team felt epitomized the co-design values expressed by workshop participants, was the 'interactive xylophone' idea. Instead of interacting with it in the same way one would do with a traditional instrument, digital technologies were employed to make a more playful and interactive experience. Interaction was facilitated in two different ways, offering park users an engaging way of exercising whilst having fun creating their own music.

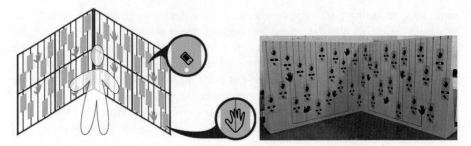

Fig. 1. The co-designed 'interactive xylophone' proof-of-concept prototype

One of the interactions allows the users to use an NFC enabled mobile phone to scan hidden RFID tags (embedded into the design) and play, note by note, 'Twinkle, Twinkle Little Star', by following the numbers displayed on the mobile phone. In order to play the tune correctly, one has to scan the correct notes as fast as possible, making it into a very challenging game. The second type of interaction allows the players to directly interface with the 'interactive xylophone' by placing and holding one hand on the large painted hand, and with the other free hand, touch any of the other smaller hands scattered around the 'interactive xylophone' (all hands are painted using conductive paint). Because it uses conductive technology multiple players can engage at the same time provided there is a physical connection between them.

5 Preliminary Results and Discussion

The 'interactive xylophone' proof-of-concept prototype was tested in the park during a community event in late June 2014. Over 150 visitors across different ages interacted with it during the day. Users left written feedback on our 'Graffiti Walls' commenting on what they liked the most about it and how it could be improved. Video observations and informal discussion were also made with several users.

Feedback, generating a number of interesting points was gathered from the pilot testing in the park. Firstly, it was evident that playfulness is ageless. People across all age groups were interacting together, learning from each other and having fun. The artefact provides a focus for intergenerational bridging, which directly relates to the participants stated values. Playful interactions aimed at public health and exercise in public spaces could offer significant benefits to park users. Developing this approach would facilitate connectedness between people and across different ages.

There are fun ways of keeping active and playfulness is a key in engaging sedentary people in casual physical activity. When the exercises are incorporated (made transparent) within a playful environment (an interactive toy or game) we noticed people increasing their physical exertion. Such experiences can be made more enjoyable through multisensorial interactions that involve touch, audio and vision, such as the 'interactive xylophone'. Having artefacts designed at a large scale is important in order to facilitate and encourage moment and physical exertion.

6   Conclusion and Future Work

We were most encouraged by the public reaction to exercising in a playful manner while using the 'interactive xylophone'. The interaction mode through the conductive technology received a lot more attention and was seen as a more natural way of inter- action. Although the mobile interaction mode allows for easier incorporation of games there are issues around accessibility. The most interesting element of the 'in- teractive xylophone' was that concepts such as this encourage grandparents and grandchildren to interact together, bridging in this way the generation gap.

We are currently in the process of redesigning it based on the feedback received, focusing more on playful aspects of the conductive mode of interaction. We are look- ing at concepts that gamify it further with a focus on the multiplayer interaction, in order to conduct more pilots with the public and collect more feedback on its playful and physical exertion aspects. We also plan to conduct a pilot with our NHS partner to investigate the health outcomes of such interventions for public health.

7   Acknowledgements

We thank all community members and our funders, the FASS-Enterprise Centre and the Catalyst research project at Lancaster University, funded by the EPSRC.

8   References

[1] OpenSpace (2010) Research Report: Community green: using local spaces to tackle inequality and improve health. http://www.openspace.eca.ac.uk/

[2] Walsh R, Boberg M, Arrasvuori J, et al. (2010) Introducing game and playful experiences to other application domains through personality and motivation models. 2010 2nd Int IEEE Consum Electron Soc Games Innov Conf 1–8.

[3] Iguchi K, Inakage M (2006) Morel: remotely launchable outdoor playthings. Proc. 2006 ACM SIGCHI

[4] Rashid O, Bamford W, Coulton P (2006) PAC-LAN□: Mixed-Reality Gaming with RFID- Enabled Mobile Phones. 4:1–17.

[5] Vogiazou Y, Raijmakers B, Geelhoed E, et al. (2006) Design for emergence: experiments with a mixed reality urban playground game. Pers Ubiquitous Comput 11:45–58.

[6] Romero N, Sturm J, Bekker T, et al. (2010) Playful persuasion to support older adults' social and physical activities. Interact Comput 22:485–495.

[7] Bekker, T., Surm, J., Eggen, B. (2010) Designing playful interactions for social interaction and physical play. Personal and Ubiquitous Computing Journal. 14. 385-396

[8] Sanders EB-N, Stappers PJ (2008) Co-creation and the new landscapes of design. CoDesign 4:5–18.

Changamoto: Design and Validation of a Therapy Adherence Game

Katinka van der Kooij[1], Evert Hoogendoorn[2], Renske Spijkerman[3], Valentijn Visch[1]

[1]Technische Universiteit Delft, Faculty of Industrial Design Engineering, Delft,
The Netherlands
[2]IJsfontein, Amsterdam, The Netherlands
[3]Parnassia Addiction Research Centre (PARC), Brijder Addiction Care, The Hague,
The Netherlands

Abstract. In the Changamoto world, Droids battle against hostile Aliens, slowly discovering which types can be easily beaten and which require more experience. The Droids are being controlled by Jeffrey, one of the thousands of Dutch youngsters that receive therapy for cannabis addiction. While Jeffrey trains his Droids and learns to strategically stage them against the right Aliens, he reminds himself to register his triggers for cannabis use in a diary.

Keywords: Gamification, therapy-adherence, cognitive behavioral therapy

1   Introduction

In this paper we set out the reasoning behind the Changamoto story and describe the validation study that will provide insight into the contribution of a serious game in therapy for cannabis addiction. Over the past decade a growing number of youngsters has been treated for cannabis addiction (Nationale drugsmonitor, 2011). In the Netherlands, a common treatment for adolescent cannabis addiction is outpatient cognitive behavioral therapy (CBT), which takes about 6 months and is generally delivered by individual face-to-face sessions with a therapist. In addition, youngsters receive therapy assignments that they have to fulfill at home. An important aspect of these assignments is registration of triggers for cannabis use. This registration provides insight in the chain of events and cognitive reactions that precedes use, and sets the groundwork for effective self-control strategies. Adherence to such homework assignments is important for gaining beneficial CBT outcomes [1,2], but problematic for youngsters receiving therapy for addiction [3].

Therapy adherence can be stimulated by providing (financial) rewards [4,5]. Providing rewards is controversial however: they could undermine intrinsic motivation [6,7,8]. Moreover, in an age of cuts on healthcare budgets, resources for providing such rewards are limited. In the G-motiv project, the game designers of IJsfontein, psychologists of Brijder Addiction Care and design researchers of the TU Delft have joined forces to explore the possibilities of using games as a self-replenishing source of rewards that do not interfere with intrinsic motivation. We spoke to patients and therapists, performed user studies and prototype tests. In this paper, we introduce the design vision and validation study of the resulting Changamoto game. We describe our design and validation study in a general Persuasive Game Design (PGD, [9; Figure 1]) framework. This way, we provide a common language that allows the formation of general guidelines on the design of persuasive games [10](also called 'serious games' [11]).

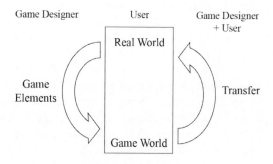

Figure 1. PGD model

2 Real-World Context

A first step in the design of a persuasive game is the definition of the real world elements that are integrated in the game design. To achieve a maximal impact on therapy adherence, we sought for the therapy component that to patients was the most relevant one and for which adherence was fundamental but at the same time practically problematic. The CBT diary to register triggers for cannabis use best suited these real-world element requirements. Addiction-focused CBT relies on the development of insight into the -often unconscious- chain of behaviors and cognitive reactions that predict the addictive behavior. Because patients see their therapists only once a week and memories fade easily, an important tool for bringing the cognitive-behavioral chain to consciousness is registration of triggers for drug use in a CBT diary. This diary teaches the patient to discriminate between external triggers (people, events and places) and internal triggers (thoughts, emotions and bodily sensations), so that they can learn how to change their behavior most effectively. Therapists indicated that adherence to this diary was often problematic: youngsters have other things on their minds than filling in a diary. Moreover the tools for diary registration weren't aligned to the context of use: the paper workbook and PC-based digital tool often were not available at the moment patients experienced their triggers. Because the CBT diary was both fundamental to therapy and could profit maximally from therapy adherence, we decided to design a game onto the real world element of the CBT diary. To enable data linkage between diary and game, we developed a new CBT diary in the form of a smartphone app.

145

3   Gamification and Game World Experience

Once the real world elements are selected, persuasive game design relies on the application of motivating game elements onto these elements [9]. In our case, we wanted to stimulate adherence to the CBT diary during the many months that therapy may take and wanted to evoke adherence even at moments when patients did not want to think about therapy. Therefore enduring motivational value and independence of motivation for therapy were the critical game-element criteria. In addition, this motivational value needed to be achieved within a budget.

The feature of enduring motivational value is created most effectively by searching her replenishing source in a combination of game rules and player development: a strategic game such as a game of chess can be played endlessly whereas an adventure game looses its motivational power once it has been completed. Therefore we chose strategy as our primary game element. From a psychological perspective, games are motivating because they feed the psychological needs of autonomy, competence and relatedness [12,13]. Here, we focused solely on autonomy and competence and not on relatedness, since interaction with peers in the delicate context of therapy can be risky because of privacy concerns. To feed the psychological needs of autonomy and competence, we chose strategy (freedom of choice), rewards and a balanced virtual opponent as our primary game elements. A combination of playtests with the user group and simulations with the game rules allowed us to check the game balancing.

To address the second game-element requirement of independence of therapeutic content, we chose an abstract narrative of different types of Droids fighting against Aliens. The narrative does not include overt references to therapy for cannabis addiction but, on an implicit level, does serve as a metaphor for the therapeutic process in which patients connect with their strengths and weaknesses, learning to optimally deal with their triggers for cannabis use. Along the same rationale, the visual design of the Droids and Aliens is minimalistic and cartoonish, yet does contain references to character traits common among addicts (i.e. a fire Droid that represents impulsivity). We hence came to the design of Changamoto: a strategic, turn-based game in which the player battles with a team of three Droids against three Aliens (Figure 2). The goal is to let Droids evolve by gaining experience points, which can be gained by eliminating hostile Aliens in one-to-one fights. Success in eliminating Aliens depends on strategically choosing with which type of Droid to fight which type of Alien.

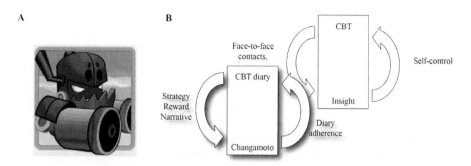

Fig. 2. A) Changamoto's fire Droid. **B)** Schematic representation of Changamoto's persuasive game design.

4   Rewards that Achieve a Transfer Effect on CBT Diary Use

The aim of Changamoto is to stimulate adherence to the CBT diary. To achieve this link between game and real world context, we reward diary entries in the game. Promoting adherence by means of rewards is controversial because the extrinsic rewards could interfere with intrinsic motivation [6, 7]. Not all rewards interfere with intrinsic motivation however [8] and there are reasons to suspect that game rewards are less prone to have negative impacts on intrinsic motivation. Performance-contingent rewards generally show less interference with intrinsic motivation than task non-contingent rewards [7, 8]. Moreover, when the reward is interpreted in relation to feelings of self-determination and competence it tends to have a more positive effect on intrinsic motivation [14]. Game rewards are delivered in a game world that is experienced as free and which fosters feelings of competence and autonomy [12]. Moreover, as most games contain direct feedback and attainable goals [11], they are suited for providing the task-contingent rewards that least interfere with intrinsic motivation.

When designing the reward of CBT diary use in Changamoto, enduring motivational value was again our primary focus. Game rewards derive their motivational value from the overarching game and therefore the motivational value of the larger game should be the primary focus. Whether a game fosters sustained engagement and positive experiences depends heavily on the balance between the challenges and successes the player encounters ('game balancing'). Successful game balancing fulfills a need for competence [12, 13], may eventually result in the highly pleasurable experience of flow [14] and sustains dramatic tension [15]. It is therefore crucial to design a game reward that provides sufficient incentives for therapy adherence but does not allow the player to be successful in the game regardless of skill. We chose to reward diary completion by unlocking extra strategic 'Swap' power upon completion of the CBT diary. By using the 'Swap' power, the player can let two Droids swap their position in a turn-taking cue. This provides strategic opportunities: a dangerous opponent can be tackled by letting a stronger Droid play first and weaker characters can gain experience before they are eliminated. The Swap power does not break the game's balancing: the reward depends on the players' skill and is no guarantee for success.

5   Validation

At the writing of this paper we have started a large randomized controlled trial (RCT), in which we aim to determine whether playing the Changamoto game increases adherence to the CBT diary (the intended transfer effect). The validation study is performed among 130 youngsters that enter therapy for cannabis addiction at Brijder Addiction Care and that have not been diagnosed with game addiction.

To measure to effect of the Changamoto game on therapy adherence, we created two conditions: a Baseline condition in which patients receive only the CBT diary from the Changamoto app and a Game condition in which subjects receive the full Changamoto app including the diary and the game. In a between-subjects design we randomly assigned the patients of each practitioner to either a baseline or a game condition. Following randomization we use the Changamoto app to track each patient's therapy adherence and –when assigned to the Game condition- play behavior for a two-month period. Therapy adherence is measured by the number of entries in the CBT diary and play behavior is measured by recordings of game choices and play duration. At the end of the two-month period we can determine whether the Changamoto game increased therapy adherence by comparing the total number of diary entries in the baseline and game condition.

Moreover, by studying the relation between play behavior, user experiences and diary entries we can evaluate the choices in Changamoto's game design: was the game well-balanced, did the game elements foster the experiences of competence and autonomy they were designed for and, finally, did the reward for CBT diary completion stimulate its use without interfering with intrinsic motivation? At the Games for Health Europe 2014 conference we will present the first results from the validation study based on which we will provide guidelines for other researchers.

6   References

[1] Carroll KM, Nich C, Ball SA (2005). Practice makes progress? Homework assignments and outcome in treatment of cocaine dependence. *Journal of Clinical Consulting and Psychology, 73*, 749-755.

[2] Hogue A, Dauber S, Chinchilla P, Fried A, Henderson C, Inclan J, Reiner RH, Liddle HA (2008). Assessing fidelity in individual and family therapy for adolescent substance abuse. *Journal of Substance Abuse Treatment, 35*, 137-147.

[3] Stark M (1992). Dropping out of substance abuse treatment: A clinically oriented review. *Clinical Psychology Review, 12*, 1, 93-116.

[4] Garcia-Rodriguez, O., Secades-Villa, R., Higgins, S. T., Fernandez-Hermida, J. R., Carballo, J. L., Errasti Perez, J. M., & Diaz, S. A. H. (2009). Effects of voucher-based intervention on abstinence and retention in an outpatient treatment for cocaine addiction: a randomized controlled trial. *Experimental and Clinical Psychopharmacology, 17*(3), 131-138.

[5] Haynes, R. B., McDonald, H. P., & Garg, A. X. (2002). Helping patients follow prescribed treatment: clinical applications. *Jama, 288*, 2880-2883.

[6] Deci, E. L., Koestner, R., & Ryan, R. M. (1999). A meta-analytic review of experiments examining the effects of extrinsic rewards on intrinsic motivation. *Psychological Bulletin, 125,* 627 - 668.

[7] Eisenberger, R., Pierce, W. D., & Cameron, J. (1999). Effects of reward on intrinsic motivation—Negative, neutral, and positive: Comment on Deci, Koestner, and Ryan (1999). *Review of educational research, 71,* 1-27.

[8] Cerasoli, C. P., Nicklin, J. M., & Ford, M. T. (2014). Intrinsic Motivation and Extrinsic Incentives Jointly Predict Performance: A 40-Year Meta-Analysis. *Psychological Bulletin, 140,* 980-1008.

[9] Visch VT, Vegt N, Anderiessen H, van der Kooij K (2013) Persuasive game design: a model and its definitions. *CHI conference publication, Paris.*

[10] Bogost, I. (2007). Persuasive games: The expressive power of videogames. Mit Press.

[11] Schell J. (2008). The Art of Game Design: A book of lenses. CRC Press.

[12] Ryan, R. M., Rigby, C. S., & Przybylski, A. (2006). The motivational pull of video games: A self-determination theory approach. *Motivation and Emotion, 30,* 344-360.

[13] Przybylski AK, Rigby CS, Ryan RM (2010) A motivational model of video game engagement. *Review of General Psychology, 14,* 154-166.

[14] Deci, E. L., Koestner, R., & Ryan, R. M. (1999). A meta-analytic review of experiments examining the effects of extrinsic rewards on intrinsic motivation. Psychological Bulletin, 125, 627 - 668.

[15] Csikszentmihalyi (1990) *Flow: The Psychology of Optimal Experience.* Harper & Row, New York.

[16] LeBlanc M (2006). Tools for creating dramatic game dynamics. *The game design reader: a rules of play anthology.* Edited by Salen K and Zimmerman E.

Author Index